What's a *joint* like this doing in a *nice girl* like you?

By Dan Tolva

Photos and text copyright © 2018 by Dan and Colleen Tolva

Thanks ...

... To the medical staff at the Vancouver Clinic and Salmon Creek Legacy Hospital in Vancouver, Wash., and to all the family and friends who helped our "Plucky Lass" through weeks of recuperation.

Contents

Foreword 1

A Spectacular Beginning 4

The First Rough Night 6

A Bit More Mobile 7

Putting the Pill in Pillow 8

Still Week in the Knee 9

Way Ahead of the Game 9

Machine Keeps New Knee Limber 11

Not All Sweetness and Light 12

Rough Night But Better Day 14

The Simple Joys Shower Down 16

It's Getting More Normal Around Here 17

Helping Hands Abound 18

A Fork, a Phone, What Fun! 20

What Stir Crazy Looks Like 21

Now She's Raising Cane 23

A Real Red-Letter Day 25

Pick 'Em: Pavement or Pain 28

Of Ugly Turquoise and Smelly Chicken Livers 29

Stove-top Huffing About My (Hazardous) Cooking Skills ... 32

Colleen's Tough Choice 35

Pantry Project Got My Gloat 37

The Last 'Update' 40

Springing the Surprise 42

More Positive News..45
The Gory Truth 47
The Problem With Normal..48
Winding Down, Probably...51
A Trip Up the Gorge..52
Sadness and a Little Joy..54
Happy Birthday to Me 57
The Surgeon Speaks 61
A Little Stumble 63
 Back to the Doc 66
A Word From Colleen..66
About the Author 70

What's a joint like this ...

Foreword

Being a child of the 1960s, I thought a joint-replacement clinic was a place where I could get medical marijuana. But, as I discovered via a four-month adventure with my lovely wife Colleen, joint-replacement clinics are providing an essential service to hundreds of thousands of people all over the country every year

As it turns out, according to media reports, there are more than 1 million joint-replacement surgeries each year, most of them hip and knee operations. It's estimated that within five years, 5 million people a year will get new joints

Just the idea of having a major part of your body cut out and replaced with a titanium alloy and plastic device is daunting. When we discovered that Colleen was going to need a new left knee in the summer of 2017, we realized that a critical change in lifestyle was at hand.

And so it was. Just preparing for Colleen's Aug. 29 surgery involved taking a class, finding out as much as we could about the procedure, and trying to anticipate how our lives would be changed

So, when Colleen got her new knee at the hands of Dr. Casey Cornelius, we weren't at all surprised about how our lives changed. What was unexpected, however was how enriching and positive the four-month-long experience really was.

As I told Colleen later, it would almost be worth the benefit to our relationship for me to shatter her right kneecap with a hammer just so we could go through the procedure again. I was only kidding, of course.

But there's no doubt that the experience enriched our lives. And the main reason for that was that we had plenty of help coping with the new circumstances.

First, there was the wonderful staff of doctors, therapists, and nurses at Salmon Creek Clinic and Salmon Creek Legacy hospital in Hazel Dell, just north of Vancouver, Wash. These people were supportive, concerned, and just as

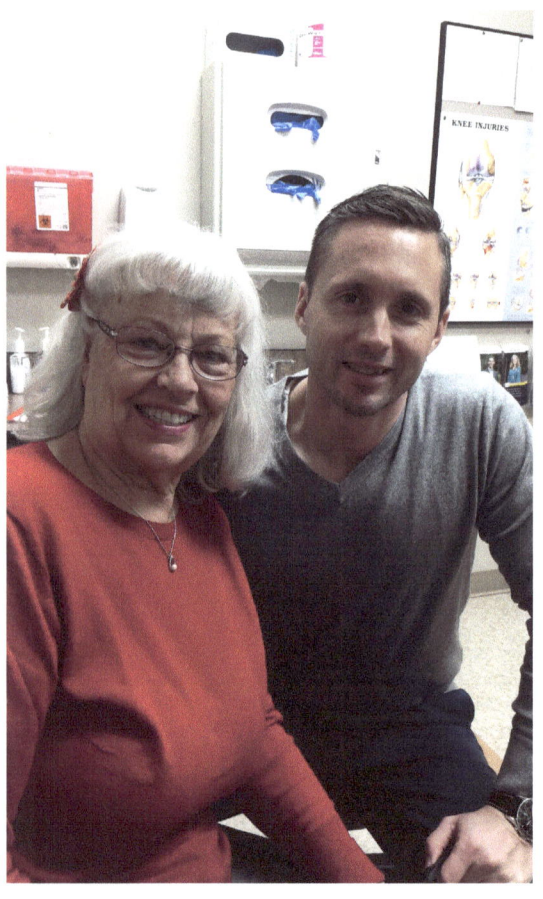

Photo by Dan Tolva

Dr. Casey Cornelius poses with one of his knee-replacement patients, Colleen Tolva, at a Dec. 4, 2017, check-up.

important, good-natured about what we were going through.

Second, we had family and friends eager to help at every turn. Colleen's son and two daughters, Kevin, Kelly, and Kasey, and Kevin's wife, Karla, we're always on hand to bring food, provide transportation, and always provide us with loving support.

And the wonderful members of our church, the Church of Jesus Christ of Latter-day Saints, were on hand without fail with food, transportation, and companionship.

Of course, all of these assets would have done little good without Colleen's enormous good cheer, faith, and optimism. For the next five months, she bubbled along, exuding joy and confidence.

That's not to say that there wasn't a lot of pain and a lot of tears along the way, because there were. But those, in a curious way provided the salt and pepper, the saver, to our experiences.

For four months or so, I documented Colleen's progress with semi-regular posts on Facebook, complete with photos and video. In November, I got the bright idea of putting all these together in a scrapbook for Colleen.

Armed with my handy iMac and the publishing software quarkXpress, I designed a 12-x 12-inch format scrapbook as a surprise gift for Colleen. The project was finished in early December, with able help of Colleen's youngest daughter, Kasey, and we presented it to her as a surprise while she was teaching a piano lesson to a young student.

Then the idea dawned on us that our experiences could benefit the many thousands of others facing the understandable fear and uncertainty of joint-replacement surgery.

"What's a Join Like This Doing in a Nice Girl Like You?" Is our offering to those who can use a little reassurance during these challenging times. We earnestly hope that our experiences can help ease the difficult experience that joint-replacement surgery offers.

— **Dan Tolva**
January 2018

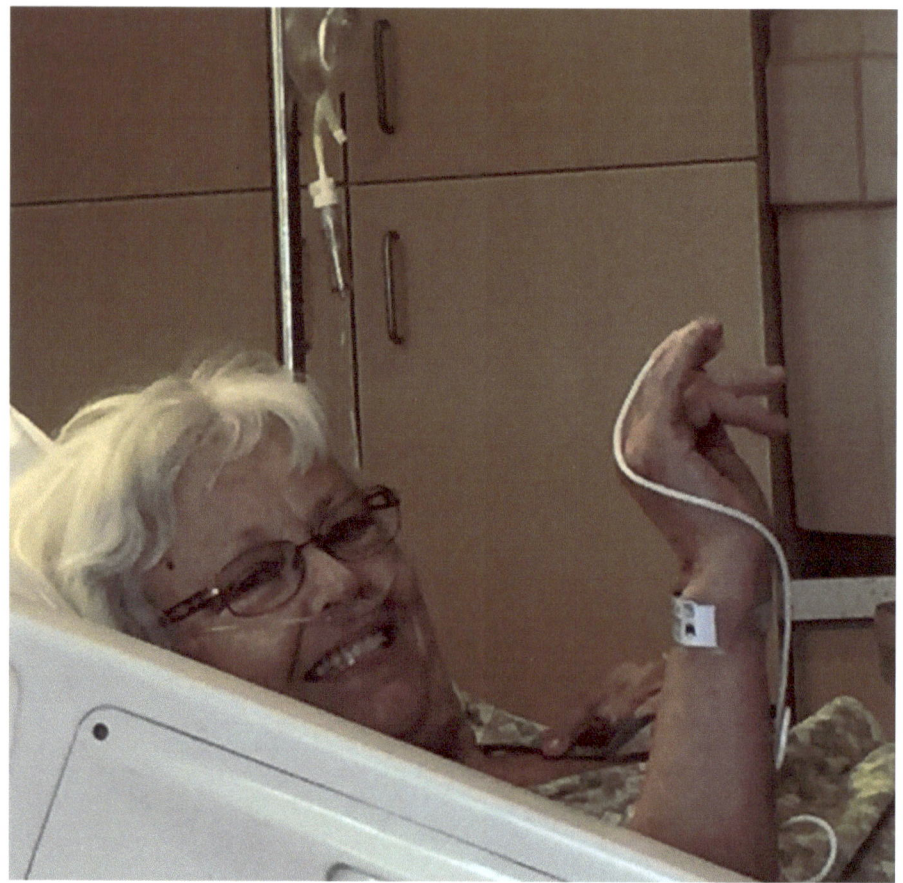

Photo by Dan Tolva

Colleen all hooked up and all smiles after surgery.

A Spectacular Beginning

Aug. 30, 2017

Colleen update: It's Wednesday, and Colleen is doing spectacularly, according to the medical staff around here.

Here is a picture of Colleen in her hospital bed, smiling. Must be the drugs.

We're expecting to go home sometime today. Thanks everybody for your kind wishes.

... Doing in a nice girl like you? 5

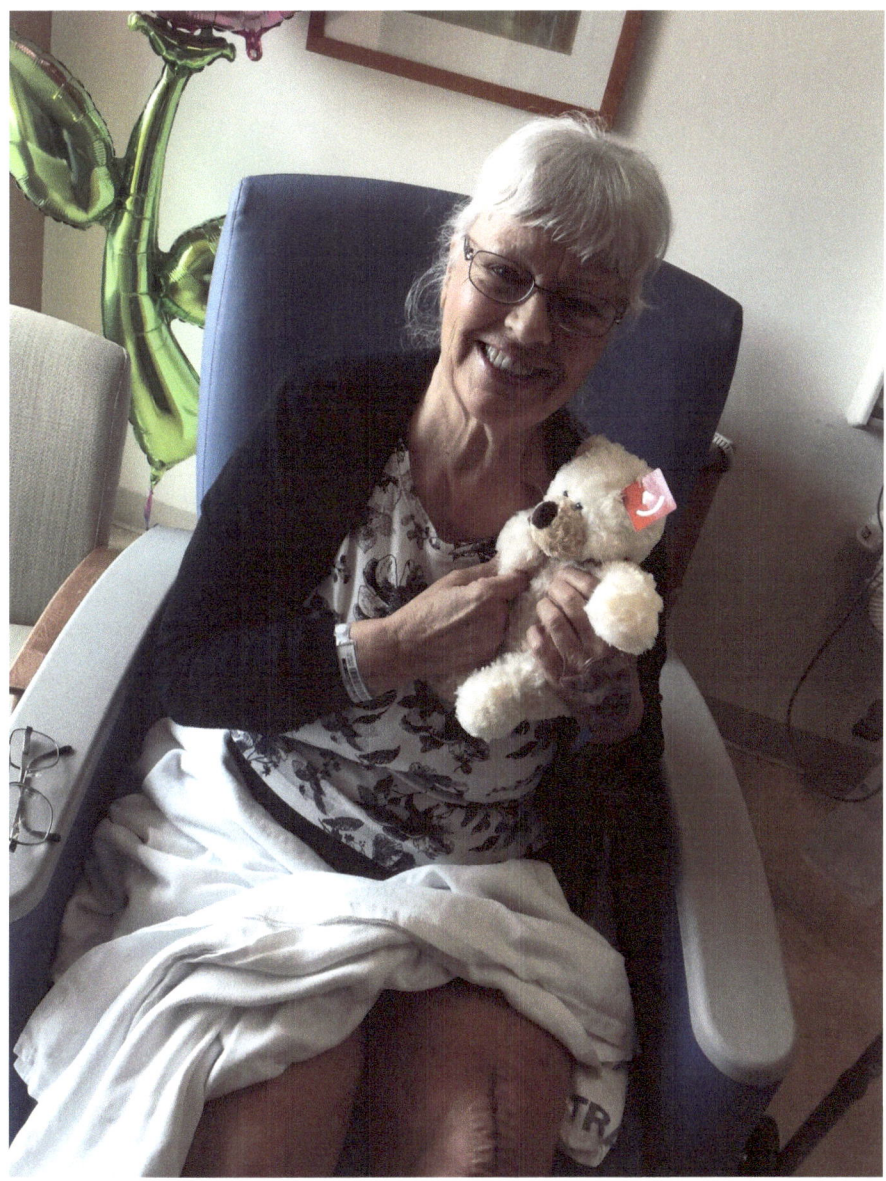

Photo by Dan Tolva
Colleen gets comfort from a fuzzy new friend and some

The First Rough Night

Aug. 31, 2017

Colleen update: Last night was pretty rough, with anesthesia finally wearing off on the new knee. Lots of pills today, but she's plugging away at her exercises, and her first physical therapy session is Friday morning.

She got outside for a short walk today, negotiating the front steps and a sloping driveway. She moans and groans a lot, but remains semi-perky.

All of your calls, visits, and prayers are appreciated and welcome. Thanks so much for your well-wishes.

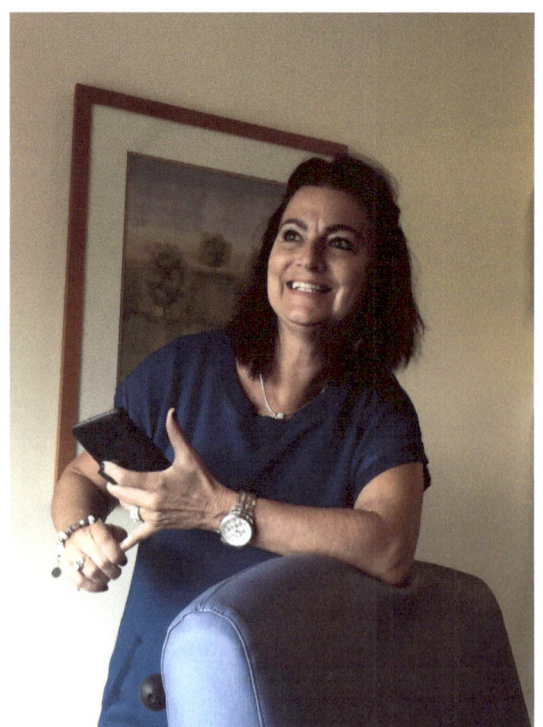

Photos by Dan Tolva

Daughter Kelly sits with Colleen in the hospital.

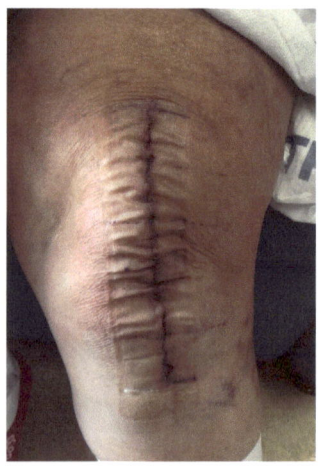

That is one nasty looking wound!

A Bit More Mobile

Sept. 2, 2017

It's Day 5 of the new knee era, and Colleen seems a bit more mobile.

We are still wrestling with medication schedules and getting enough sleep, but family members and friends have been doing so much for us, I'm sure we are getting along better than otherwise.

Everybody has been so nice, and your prayers and well wishes are greatly appreciated.

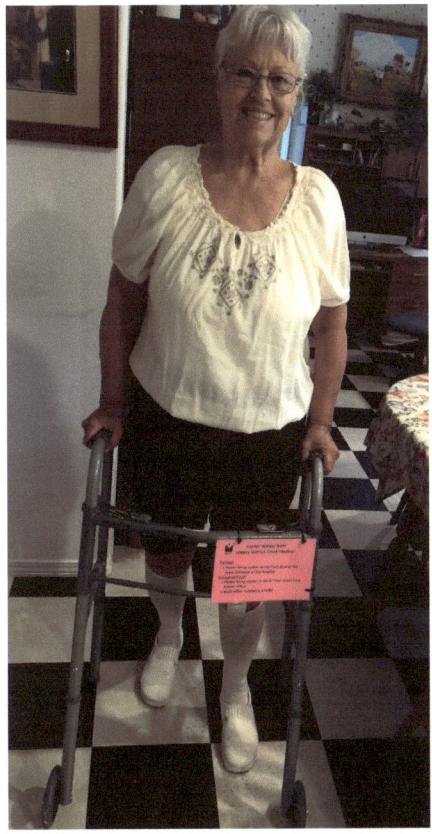 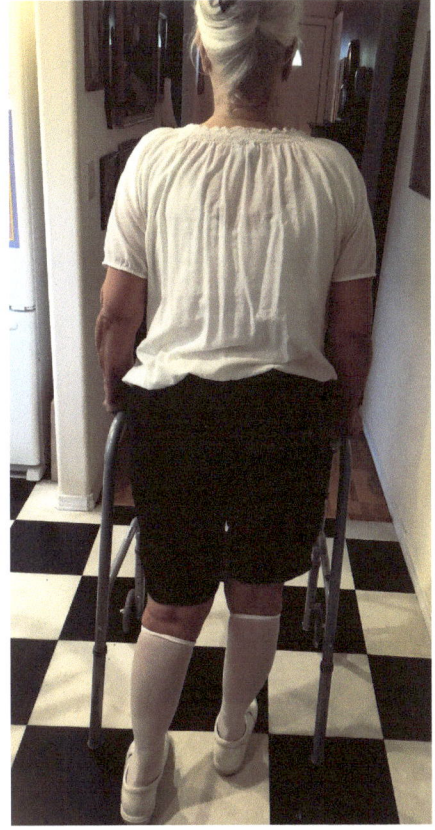

Photos by Dan Tolva

Colleen looks good coming or going.

Putting the Pill in Pillow

Sept. 3, 2017

The new knee is growing stronger but still hurts a lot. Her pill schedule wakes us up at least four times a night, but it's worth it to keep the pain in check.

Colleen is really good about doing her exercises, which consist of five sessions daily, each with about 10 different routines. She's had physical therapy once and is due for another session Tuesday. She's walking more and more, and now and then gets so gung-ho that she'll forget her walker and start out on just her own two feet.

Everybody has been so supportive, especially Colleen's kids, Kelly, Kasey, Kevin, and his wife, Karla. Their kindness, thoughtfulness, and love has made this challenge much easier to endure. Colleen thanks all of you. Me, too.

As you might expect, sleeping is an important part of Colleen's recovery plan, and she takes just about every opportunity to catch a cat nap. I do, too, for that matter.

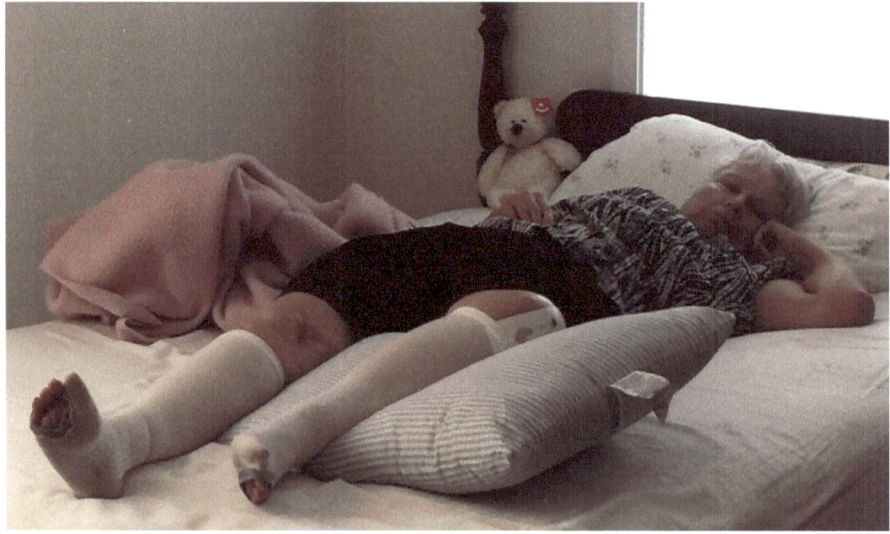

Photo by Dan Tolva

Time for a little snooze.

Still Week in the Knee

Sept. 4, 2017

Colleen update: Well, Colleen has had her replacement knee for seven days now. I guess that means she's week-kneed. Colleen has shown much improvement since last Tuesday, the day of her surgery. There's still a lot of work to do, but she's s real trooper, she is. Soon she'll be frolicking in the meadows and gamboling on the hillsides.

And gone will be the days when her doctor will look at her deformed left leg and have to ask, "What's a joint like this doing in a nice girl like you?"

Way Ahead of the Game

Sept. 7, 2017

Colleen update: Our gal is plugging away at getting her new knee stronger, with another physical therapy session today (See photo at right.). The therapist says Colleen is way ahead of most folks who get artificial knees these days.

In fact, Colleen was standing in front of the kitchen sink this morning, and her walker, though nearby, was out of sight. She looked and acted completely normal for that moment, and I forgot for an instant she was on the mend from serious surgery.

The routine is getting dull: Pill at 12:45 a.m.; pill at 3:45 a.m.; pill at 5:30 a.m.; pill at 6:45 a.m.; pill at 9:45 a.m.; pill at 11:30 a.m.; pill at 12:45 p.m.; pill at 3:45 p.m.; pill at 5:30 p.m.; pill at 6 p.m.; pill at 9:45 p.m.; and pill at 11:30 p.m.

All of her times are logged into my iPhone alarm clock, with each type of pill with its own alert sound. How geeky can I get?

It's my duty to alert her day and night as to what pill to take, and I also get to supervise her exercises and her walking. She has been outside the past few days, but her time and distance walked have been limited by the smokey air. But when the smoke finally does go away, I'm working her ragged, I tell you!

As usual, Colleen's family and friends have been wonderful about bringing in food and providing transportation to physical therapy and doctors' appointments. The car has been in the garage the past couple of weeks, thereby escaping our recent ash fall.

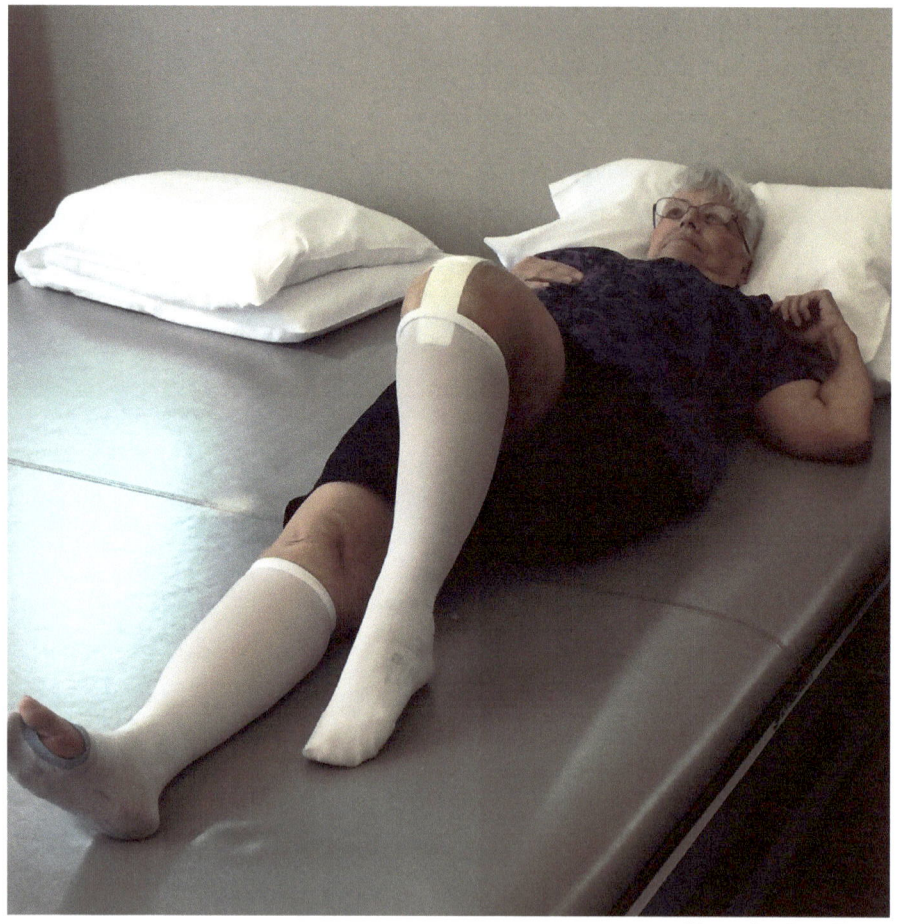

Photo by Dan Tolva

Looking good during physical therapy.

... Doing in a nice girl like you?

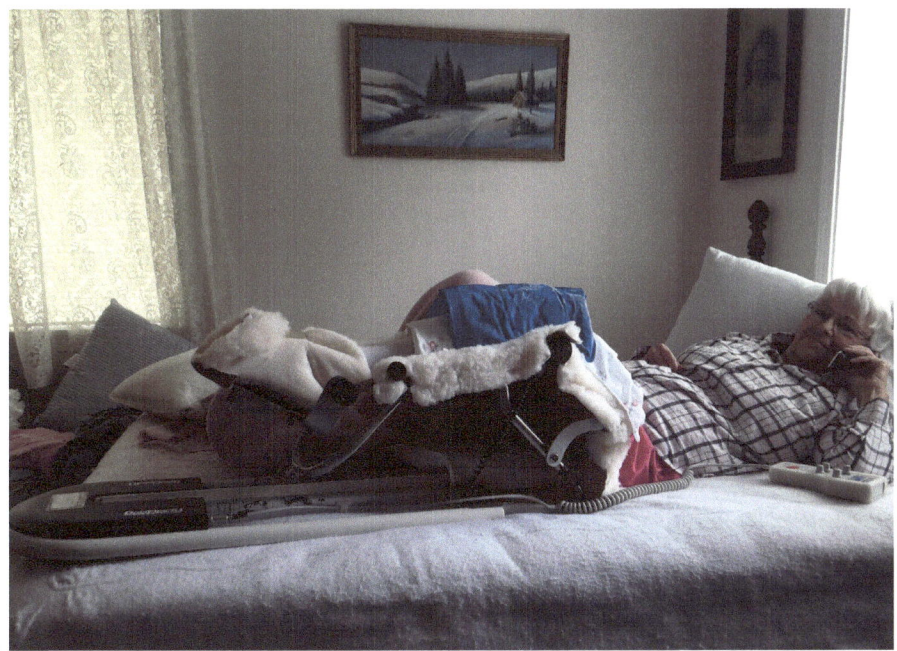

Photo by Dan Tolva

Here's Colleen and that raise-and-move-your-leg-up-and-down thingy.

Machine Keeps New Knee Limber

Sept. 8, 2017

Colleen update: Here's our plucky gal during one of her daily post-operation rituals.

That oddball looking machine is for elevating her leg with its new knee, and the machine also moves her leg to keep the knee flexible.

While using it, we ice her down with one of those blue packs we keep in the freezer. Those are handy little gadgets, and I'd like to get a couple more of them just in case Colleen and I are laid up together.

Colleen ran a couple of errands to the clinic and to the eye glasses people today, getting out both times and making the short walk from and to the van on her own. (Thanks to daughter Kasey for providing the transportation.)

Everybody who sees Colleen remarks on how chipper and energetic she seems to be. I'm sure her positive attitude and cheerful disposition have a lot to do with what seems a remarkable recovery. There's a lot more work to do, but I'm sure all will turn out fine.

Thanks to all of you for your kind wishes.

You'll note, by the way, that Colleen is on the phone in the picture on Page 9. This is her normal and natural condition, so much so that the cartilage in her left ear has morphed into the shape of a phone hook. You think I'm kidding, don't you?

Not All Sweetness and Light

Sept. 10, 2017

Colleen update: If I've suggested in my previous posts regarding our plucky girl that all was sweetness and light in her recovery from knee-replacement surgery, I apologize.

Actually: the process has been grueling and challenging for her, but her cheery and peppy disposition usually belies that fact.

The last couple of days have been a case in point. Her pain persists, and if it weren't for the Tylenol and oxycodone, I can't imagine how miserable she would really be. It has been a two-steps-forward, one-step-back process the last day or so.

Part of her recuperation has involved a lot of sleep, partly because of the drugs, I suppose, and partly because the healing process does tend to take it out of you at times. On the other hand, having to take pills 13 times a day certainly disrupts her seep patterns. Mine, too, for the matter, because I'm the official Pill Reminder and Exercise Coach.

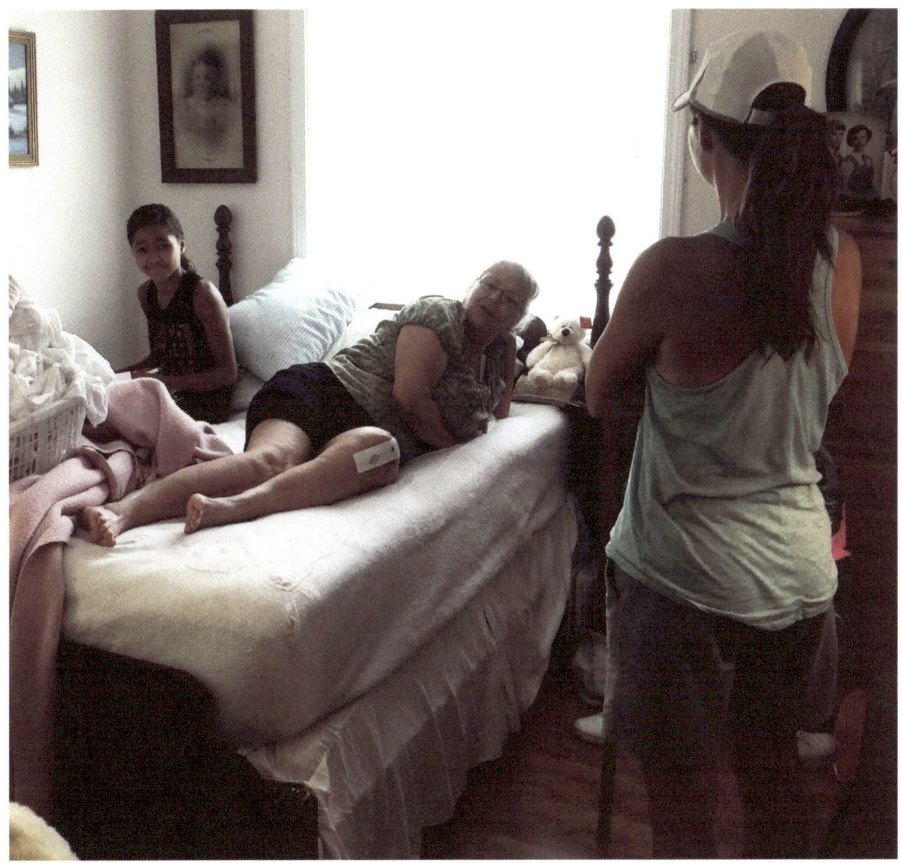

Photo by Dan Tolva

Colleen's younger daughter, Kasey, right, and granddaughter Jaden pay a visit.

(The fact that I'm posting this at 4:45 on a Sunday morning gives an idea of how disruptive the whole process has been for both of our sleep cycles.)

But as stated above, Colleen remains plucky, cheerful, determined, and extremely grateful for the support and help of many family and friends. Me, I'm just dumb and dogged, and don't know enough to be really ticked off. But I have had fun doing a lot of extra cooking, though my tendency to experiment hasn't always produced the tastiest results. (My sweet-pickle salmon rice balls come to mind.)

Monday is Colleen's first visit to the doctor since the surgery, and we're pretty sure his assessment is going to be very upbeat. So we will keep plugging along, bolstered by the good wishes of everybody out there and grateful to Heavenly Father for his healing hand in all things.

Again, thanks to all of you for your loving support, and may God bless and keep you and yours.

Rough Night But Better Day

Sept.11, 2017

Colleen update: It was another rough night for our Plucky Lass, But the new day brought a little relief from the pain and a lot of good news from the doctor.

Colleen was up in the middle of the night, crying at times, because of sharp pains just below her knee. I was there to keep her company, and so was Benny the Cat, who sat on the bed gazing fondly at his mistress and exuding tons of feline concern.

Of course I had my iPhone, which I've been using to keep track of Colleen's meds, so I turned it on and found a little soothing music: a symphony for strings by Felix Mendelssohn. The music did the trick, calming Colleen down and at least taking a little bit of the edge off the pain.

I guess from this time on I'll have to refer to old Felix as "Medicinal Mendelssohn."

The next morning we had therapy, that is, Colleen had therapy, I was just along for the ride. We learned a thing or two about how to use our ice pack. Colleen had been "double-bagging" her ice pack in two pillowcases, while the therapist used only one case for each bag, and made sure there was ice above and below the knee. The difference was amazing, Colleen said, because she could really feel the cold sink in. That in the long run should help her knee feel a lot better.

... Doing in a nice girl like you?

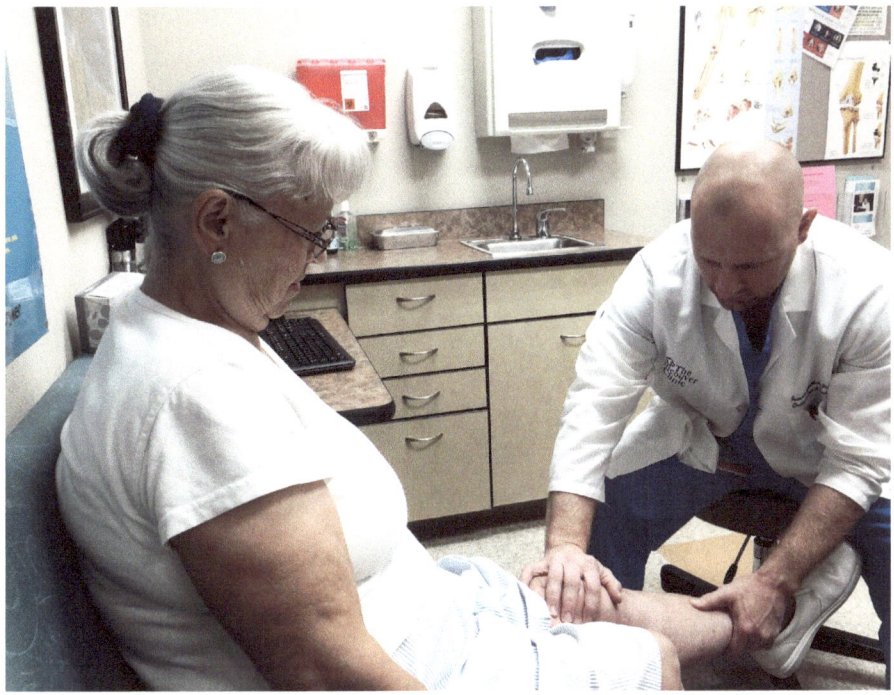

Photo by Dan Tolva

Physician's assistant Joe Mathias check's Colleen's knee.

A couple hours later, we had our first appointment with one of the medical staff who had replaced her knee. Physician's assistant Joe Mathias took off the bandage, found all was well, and said the wound could now go undressed, and that Colleen would not have to wear those extremely uncomfortable compression stockings any longer. Further, Colleen can let up on the oxycodone now, going from 12 times a day to taking it whenever she really needs it. This is really good news, because she can't drive as long as she's taking that powerful opiate, and I'm getting cabin fever. Yes, it's all about me.

After the medical appointment, Colleen and I visited a pharmacy to pick up a second ice pack and some Tylenol, then she got herself a yogurt treat at a local shop. It felt like being normal for the first time in a couple of weeks.

That, along with the wonderful weather, made the afternoon absolutely delightful. We know the challenges aren't over yet, and there probably will be a lot more pain and even a few tears along way. But at least it seems like we can see the light at the end of the tunnel.

Again we have to thank Colleen's daughter-in-law, Karla Brown, for running us all over the place and the patient, cheerful manner in which she did so. Everybody has been wonderful throughout this whole ordeal.

We're hoping now that Colleen can get a little bit more sleep at night (Me, too! Me, too!). We're also hoping that the new icing technique will help cut down the pain and swelling even more.

Thanks everybody for your prayers and well wishes. We couldn't of done it without you.

The Simple Joys Shower Down

Sept. 12, 2017

Colleen update: Oh, the simple joys of life!

With the dressing off of that nasty looking scar, our plucky lady and her new knee were able to take their first real shower in a couple of weeks. And boy, did it feel good!

(You'll excuse me for not documenting this event with a photo, as I have for recovery milestones in past posts. Let's just say that Colleen smells better, the house smells better, and her hair is squeaky clean. Her whole outlook definitely improved.)

We – I know, what's this "we" hooha – are still exercising and still walking. And we got a little help today from Colleen's visiting teachers, Sister Pam Coleman and Sister Amanda Snyder. They cleaned the kitchen and brought in a turkey dinner from Chuck's.

For those of you who don't know, the women of the Mormon Church are assigned several families to visit each month. They regularly bring service and a message of faith to all of our homes. The men have their own version of this program, known as home teaching. It's a wonderful way to minister to each other, and to help make sure that assistance from the Church is given when needed.

Speaking of service, Colleen's younger daughter, Kasey, came over and watered the flowers yesterday evening. She offered to water Benny the Cat, too, but he declined the honor. Thanks to Kasey and all of the others who have helped so much in this time of trial.

We're going to work a little more on walking over the next few days. Colleen has also made an effort to cut down on the use of oxycodone, one of her prescriptions.

As long as she's taking that powerful opiate, she won't be able to drive. And you can bet her right foot will be itching to stomp on a gas pedal.

Colleen is taking a nice little nap right now, so the house is really quiet. Just the perfect time to post an update. More physical therapy in store tomorrow.

Again, we can't thank all of you enough for your support, love, good wishes, and service.

You will be rewarded in a future life.

It's Getting More Normal Around Here

Sept. 13, 2017

Colleen update: Well, things are looking more normal day by day.

Colleen actually had breakfast at the kitchen table today after taking a shower all on her own. She also put on long pants, socks, and tennis shoes for the first time in weeks, also all on her own.

If it weren't for the walker protruding from her hands, you might think she was normal. That's assuming she is normal when she's normal. Which she isn't.

We had physical therapy again today, and Colleen continues to improve. They put her on a machine of some sort, and she enjoyed the heck out of that. Kind of like driving the car except she wasn't going anywhere, thank goodness.

In the walking department, Colleen is making great strides you might say. She went outside yesterday and made it eight driveways down before having to turn back.

One of the things I keep having to point out to her when she's walking is to keep her butt in, underneath her center of gravity.

"Butt in! Butt in!" I exhort in my best drill sergeant voice. I say it so often, Colleen's accusing me of being a butt-in-ski. Ha ha ha.

Helping Hands Abound

Sept. 14, 2017

Colleen update: A lot of people have combined to help ease Colleen's recovery from knee replacement surgery. Every day, we see another example of one generous spirit or another reaching out a hand to help.

Last night, it was Colleen's oldest daughter, Kelly, and granddaughter, Jessica, who came to the rescue. First, they picked up a special brand of Tylenol for Colleen, then they went and got us a pizza from Papa Murphy's. Then they had to go back out again and get a different kind of Tylenol. All was done with gracious and beautiful smiles.

Then there's Marianne, nicknamed Dover, one of Colleen's best friends. Dover came over and took my grandson, Liam and I shopping at WinCo for a long list of groceries. Believe me, it looked more like Larry Moe and Curly shopping, rather than Dan, Dover, and Liam. Amazingly, all the groceries were safely gathered in and put away.

And there's another friend I have to tell you about, except this one isn't

... Doing in a nice girl like you? 19

human. It's my iPhone 6.

I've had this for about a year, but so far I've only used it mostly for calls and for looking up the weather forecast. At the end of each day, the little green battery at the top of the screen was still filled, connoting plenty of power. But these days, I found so many uses for the phone that the battery is almost completely gone now at the end of each day.

Right after her surgery, Colleen had a very complicated regimen when it came to meds. She had to take oxycodone every three hours, Tylenol every six hours, and Coumadin once a day. After a few fits and starts, I discovered I could use the iPhone clock to set alarms for each pill at the appropriate hour. Each medication even had its own alert sound and label, so it was easy to tell at a glance and a listen as to what needed to be taken when. I also use the clock's stopwatch feature to time how long to leave Colleen's ice packs on. The limit is 20 minutes, by the way, unless she wants to risk freezer burn.

As I had to do the shopping now, lacking Colleen's knowledge of where things were at WinCo, I found iPhone really handy for making out our grocery list. I could add to the list as I went along, and when I was confused about brands, I could take pictures, for example of the cat food (we have a very finicky cat), and attach them to the grocery list growing on the iPhone.

I've also discovered that iPhone is great for taking dictation. These Colleen updates I've basically been dictating on the iPhone and e-mailed to myself, or I can edit them more closely and eventually post them. I've also used the iPhone to take photos and a video for these updates.

I like to think God was having an awfully good day when he invented M&Ms, Oreo cookies, and iPhones. I know, Steve Jobs gets the credit for the iPhone. But we believe all great inspiration comes directly from Heavenly Father.

Well, I just got the kitchen cleaned up from breakfast (crepes stuffed with homemade butterscotch pudding and fresh strawberries, and topped with real whipped cream), and I'm ready to hop in the shower. Again I want to thank all of those who have helped – gals, guys, and gizmos.

A Fork, a Phone, What Fun!

Sept. 15, 2017

Colleen update: A phone in one hand and a fork in the other. Can life get any better for our Plucky Lass? So what if she had to give up her real knee and endure several weeks of painful recovery. It's the good things in life that matter, as illustrated in the photo at left. The breakfast, by the way, was blueberry pancakes, eggs over easy, and apple juice. It's No. 2 on the Tolva Freehold's Extreme Seniors Menu.

Slowly but surely, Colleen is doing better. She went on two walks yesterday, one with her grandson, Liam. She was up and about much of the day, and she even fixed dinner for us last night, because I was dead to the world sleeping.

A milestone today, Colleen played the piano for the first time since before

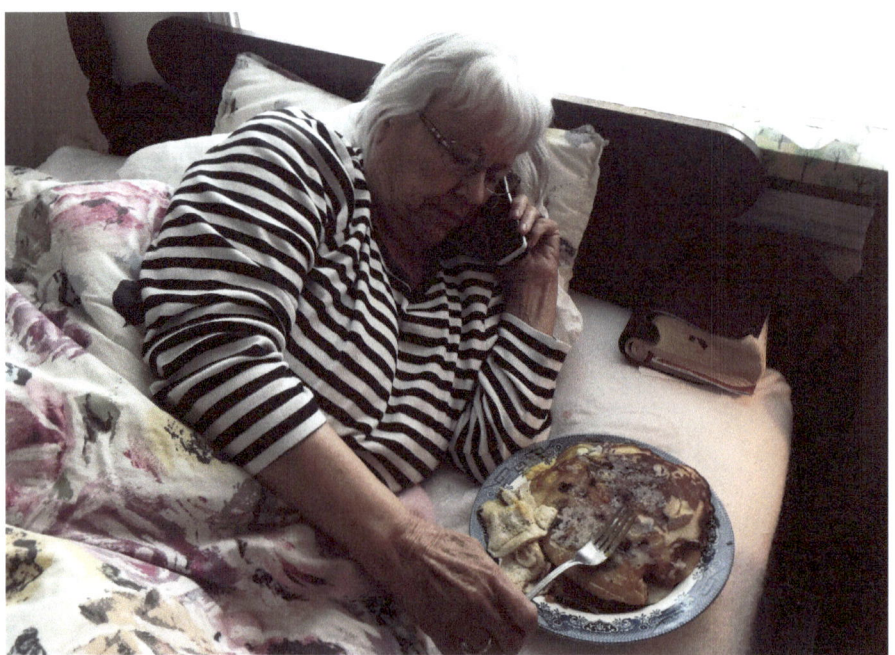

Photo by Dan Tolva

Breakfast in bed while on the phone.

her surgery. She sounded good, but felt awful. Even so she only needed to use her right foot for the petals, her left foot (site of the new knee) was at an angle calculated to bring pain. So the song didn't last long, but it was fun for her while it lasted.

Colleen went to physical therapy by herself today, because I had to stick around the house while the window washer came and did the outside windows. Colleen reports that the torture master really ran her ragged today, hurting her knee a lot, abusing her, and leaving a wreck, shattered physically and mentally.

She might be exaggerating. But the therapist did tell Colleen she probably overdid it the day before. As a result, Colleen is pretty much horizontal and unconscious right now. That's the way I'm going to be as soon as I get the kitchen cleaned up from lunch.

And I know it sounds like a broken record, but thanks, thanks, thanks for all of you who have helped with your deeds and with your prayers. That includes Karla Brown, who provided transportation to and from physical therapy today, and Ramie Scukanec, who brought over a plate of bran muffins.

What Stir Crazy Looks Like

Sept. 17, 2017

Colleen update: Examine the two photos on the next page. Experts in war injuries will tell you that both of these pictures show all the signs of combat fatigue and severe shell-shock.

This is Colleen and me after three weeks of basically staring at each other through forced togetherness. Her long convalescence from her knee replacement surgery has made it mandatory for us to stay in the same house together with virtually no break since Aug. 29. The wear and tear is beginning to show. We're looking at each other funny with long periods of silence. In simple terms, we're going stir crazy.

Oh, we're still pleasant enough to each other, on the surface, but you can

22   What's a joint like this ...

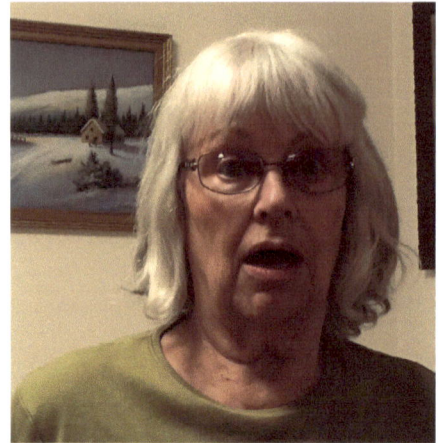 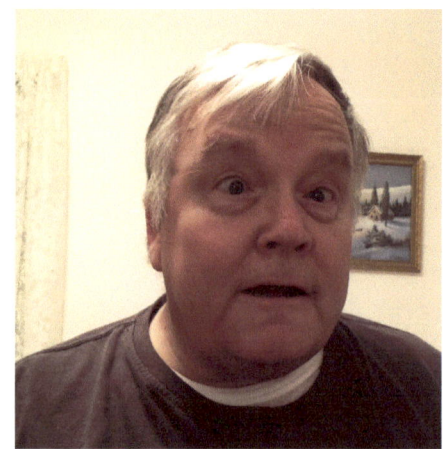

Her in shock ...   **... Me in shock**

see the jaws clenched and hear the teeth grinding at times as we try not to kill each other too much.

One thing that's helped us cope is good food. It's no accident but people on long submarine duty get a big morale boost on their gruelling tours through good food. Consequently, we really tried to eat well.

I've been doing all the cooking, and I've really tried to have a tasty variety of foods. Yesterday and today, for example, we had a nice turkey dinner with mashed potatoes and gravy, a fresh salad of onions, tomatoes and cucumbers, and canned whole-kernel corn. I'm afraid that if we would've just had peanut butter sandwiches, we would have been at each other's throats with dull, rusty knives.

Actually, it's been going really well. Colleen is working hard at her exercise and strengthening the muscles around her new knee. And we've also been bolstered by the rain Sunday, with the freshness in the air giving us a funny kind of new energy. And, of course, we've had plenty of visits and phone calls from family and friends offering encouragement and support.

Tomorrow, Monday, we have physical therapy again. But the big news is that in the afternoon, Colleen will resume teaching piano and violin. Another touch of normalcy, and fortunately another break from just staring at each other.

Now She's Raising Cane

Sept.18, 2017

Colleen update: Well, today you can mark a step up for our Plucky Lassie, and then a step down; and then a step up; and then a step down…

That little stairstepping exercise was part of colleen's physical therapy this morning. But the big news may well of been that she is transitioning from a walker to a cane.

She seems to be really keen for the cane, simply because it's not nearly as cumbersome as the walker, lightweight though it may be. She proved the value of the cane after physical therapy today by getting out of the car on her own and dashing – well, after a fashion – into a local grocery store for a few veggies. Oh, I bet you she felt independent!

(Thanks to Karla Brown again for transportation to and from physical therapy.)

You can imagine that after all that exercise Colleen was pretty darned sore when she got home. So we iced her up, and she took a short snooze while yours truly made mischief in the kitchen.

On the menu today is tuna casserole, doctored up Tolva style: Lots of mozzarella and cheddar cheese, lots of onions, lots of mushrooms, lots of cream of mushroom soup, a dollop or two of sour cream, all topped with bread crumbs mixed with melted margarine and Parmesan cheese.

This is one of those comfort dishes that one shouldn't have more than once a month, but I'm sure we're going to have leftovers tomorrow, which will be two times in September, and who knows what will be left over on Wednesday.

Colleen is looking forward to her first music students in three weeks this afternoon. She's got a comfy chair all picked out from which to monitor the budding young musicians. I hope all goes well.

As I'm finishing up this post, Colleen is in on her bed, writing in her journal.

She is an extremely prolific journal keeper. Since the 1970s she has composed enough material to fill dozens of three ring binders. As for me, Facebook has become my journal over the past few years.

Colleen tells me that if our house catches fire, she'll save the journals and leave me to fend for myself. I don't think she's joking.

It's time to sign off, but you know I can't get away with one of these posts without thanking all of you for your prayers, your good wishes, and all of your help. God bless you all.

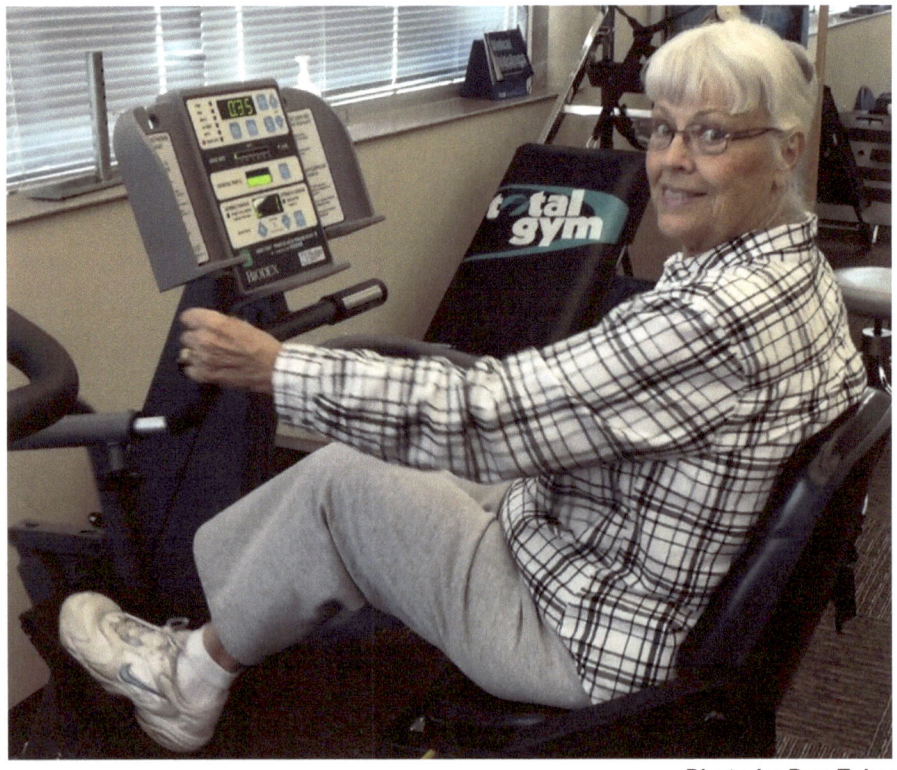

Photo by Dan Tolva

Colleen's new knee gets workout on exercise machine.

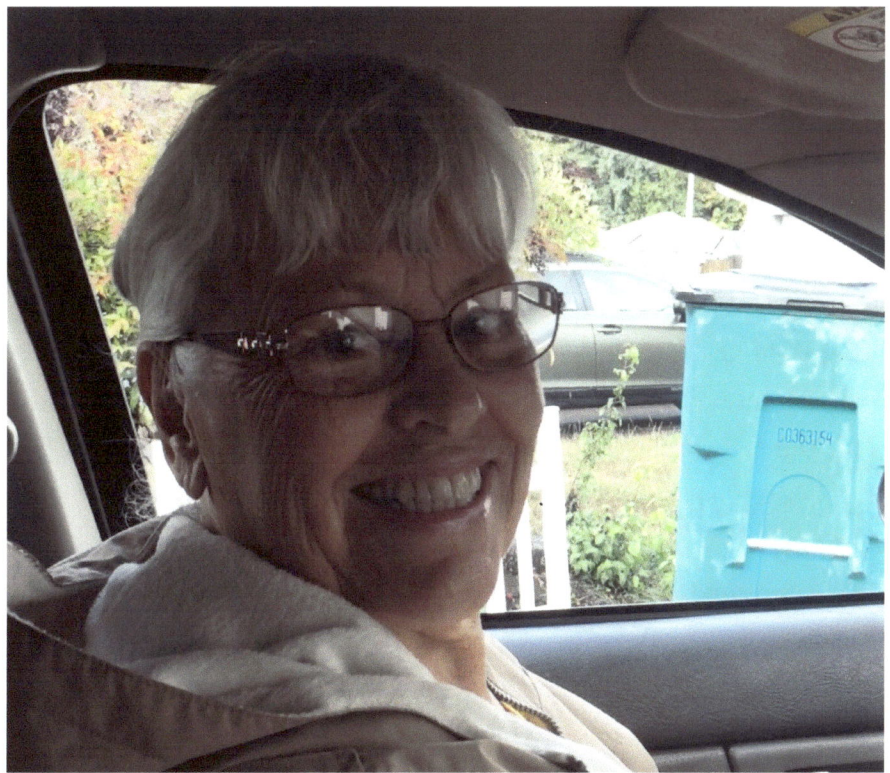

Photo by Dan Tolva

Colleen at the wheel: Look out, world!!!

A Real Red-Letter Day

Sept. 20, 2017

Colleen update: It has been three weeks and a day since our Plucky Lass got her new knee, and she continues to make great progress.

This has been a red-letter day, as Colleen marches closer and closer to full recovery. Well, not march, exactly, but kind of a stiff and stilted walk.

Yet already that walk is a much healthier looking gait than before she got her new knee. Colleen's left leg is relatively straight, not at the catawampous angle it was before the surgery, and she isn't limping.

Today at physical therapy, Colleen inched closer to a couple of milestones.

First, by using straps, Colleen was able to bend her knee backwards at a 119° angle. The goal is 120°. Then the therapist straightened out Colleen's leg and pressed on the kneecap to see how flat to the ground the leg would come. The perfect alignment is 0°, and Colleen managed 1°. The therapist was impressed.

The second really neat thing that happened today was that, with Colleen's able assistance, I made a Gravenstein apple pie from scratch. (First I scratched myself, then I started cooking.)

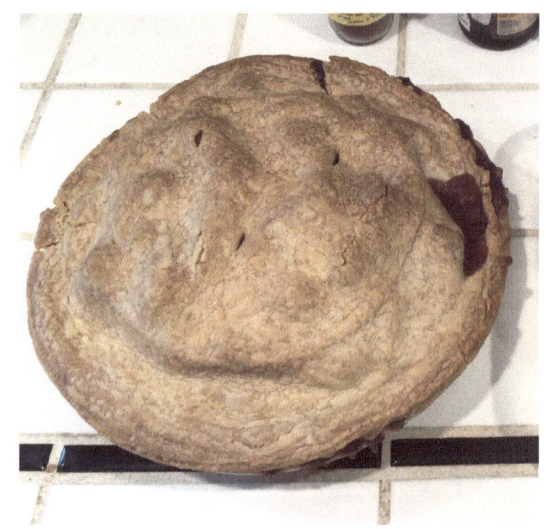

Photo by Dan Tolva

Gravenstein apple pie: Mmmmmmmm!

Any pie aficionado will tell you, or should tell you, the Gravensteins make the greatest apple pie. I cheated by using a frozen crust, but I countered with a homemade filling to die for. Colleen peeled, cored, and sliced up all the apples, which came from a tree in our backyard, and I did the rest. The pie plus a little leftover filling in a separate baking pan are cooling on the counter right now, just waiting for us to dig in.

Colleen allows as to how whipped cream would be perfect with this pie, but unfortunately, we don't have any. But Colleen has a strategy in mind to get some, and this promises to be the capper to our red-letter day. I'll tell you about it after it happens.…

… Well, it happened. The only thing preventing Colleen from getting behind the wheel of our car was the oxycodone she's been taking. But she's been cutting way down on that strong opiate, and it has been at least nine hours since she had a pill. That, according to our pharmacist, is enough time to safely drive.

So this evening, during a break teaching piano students, Colleen wedged herself into the car, started it up, and gingerly backed out of the garage. It's the first time the car has been out since Aug. 28, the day before Colleen's surgery. The vehicle has been in the garage all this time, safe from our recent ash fall and protected from the downpours of the last few days.

The outing was a short one. Colleen drove down to the mailbox, where I got the mail. Then we went down to the Corner Market, at Highway 99 and 104th Street, and bought some Reddi Whip. OK, it wasn't real whipped cream, but it'll do in a pinch.

After just a few minutes driving, Colleen's left leg started aching. So we headed back home and she eased the car into the garage. I'm sure we won't be taking any long cross-country trips anytime soon, but maybe we can make it to Church Sunday. It was just so nice to get out of the house.

So things are getting back to normal. In fact, I saw Colleen standing at the sink today and thought for sure she was going to wash a few dishes. I've already told her that once she washes her first dish, all special treatment ends, along with the breakfasts in bed, and all the pampering. Maybe that's why she declined to wash anything today. I may have doomed myself to being on permanent kitchen patrol with that rather dumb ultimatum. We'll see.

Here I need to add the names of my younger daughter, Megan, and her son, Liam, to the list of all of those who've been so wonderful about helping out.

Megan has taken me to the store and to the bank, swept and mopped the floor, and done dishes. Not to mention the fact that she and Colleen gab like a couple of teenage girls. Liam has trotted down to the mailbox almost every afternoon, and he has accompanied Colleen on some of her walks. The help sure is welcome.

Also welcome are the continued well wishes and prayers of all of you. Thank you so much.

What's a joint like this ...

Pick 'Em: Pavement or Pain

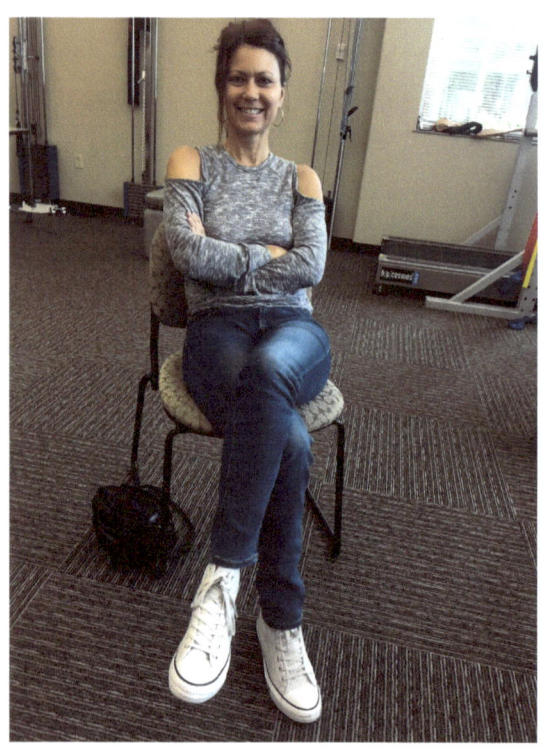

Photo by Dan Tolva

Colleen's younger daughter, Kasey Frazier, watches Mom undergo physical therapy.

Sept. 22, 2017

Colleen update: Right now, our Plucky Lass is torn between the desire to drive and the equally potent need to be as free of pain as possible.

One of the most effective ways of battling pain is to take the powerful opiate oxycodone regularly. Colleen's doctors recommend one pill every four hours, though she has been trying to cut down on its use. But as long as she's taking the pill, she can't drive for at least six to eight hours.

Otherwise, things are slowly getting back to normal. Colleen taught almost her full complement of piano and violin students this week, spending a lot of time in a reclining chair with her knee up, sometimes with ice on it.

She had another round of physical therapy today, and this time we had Colleen's youngest daughter, Kasey, to thank for transportation. A quick note hear about Colleen's physical therapy guru, Ali Jakobowski, who has been more than wonderful. A little on the tough side, too. But that's just exactly what Colleen needs right now.

After the therapy, we stopped to pick up a few groceries, then Colleen and Kasey decided to hit a local garage sale. Talk about things getting back to normal

Yours truly is still doing the cooking and KP, with a big por of old-fashioned navy beans and bacon on the menu today. I made enough to freeze a bunch, as well as provide Kasey and her family with a healthy dose. I hope they like them.

Somehow I think the next couple of weeks are going to be the toughest for Colleen, simply because it's so tempting to go back to the way things were before her knee-replacement surgery. That means it's awfully tempting to walk around without her cane, and to think that she can do everything the way she did beforehand.

But there is still a lot of pain to overcome, and a lot more work is going to be needed to strengthen the muscles around that new knee. But I'm confident that Colleen, armed with her natural happy and cheery disposition and the prayers and deeds of so many family and friends, will prevail.

Then maybe she can do the dishes again.

Of Ugly Turquoise and Smelly Chicken Livers

Sept. 24, 2017

Colleen update: The really exasperating thing about getting back to normal is that if the least little thing goes wrong, you're not back to normal. It only seems that way.

That's pretty much the way it is with Colleen at the moment. With her new knee, she can walk with good form, straight up, no limp, and by the looks of it, no pain. But scratch the surface, and you uncover a lot of discomfort.

So even though everybody's complementing her on how much better she

What's a joint like this ...

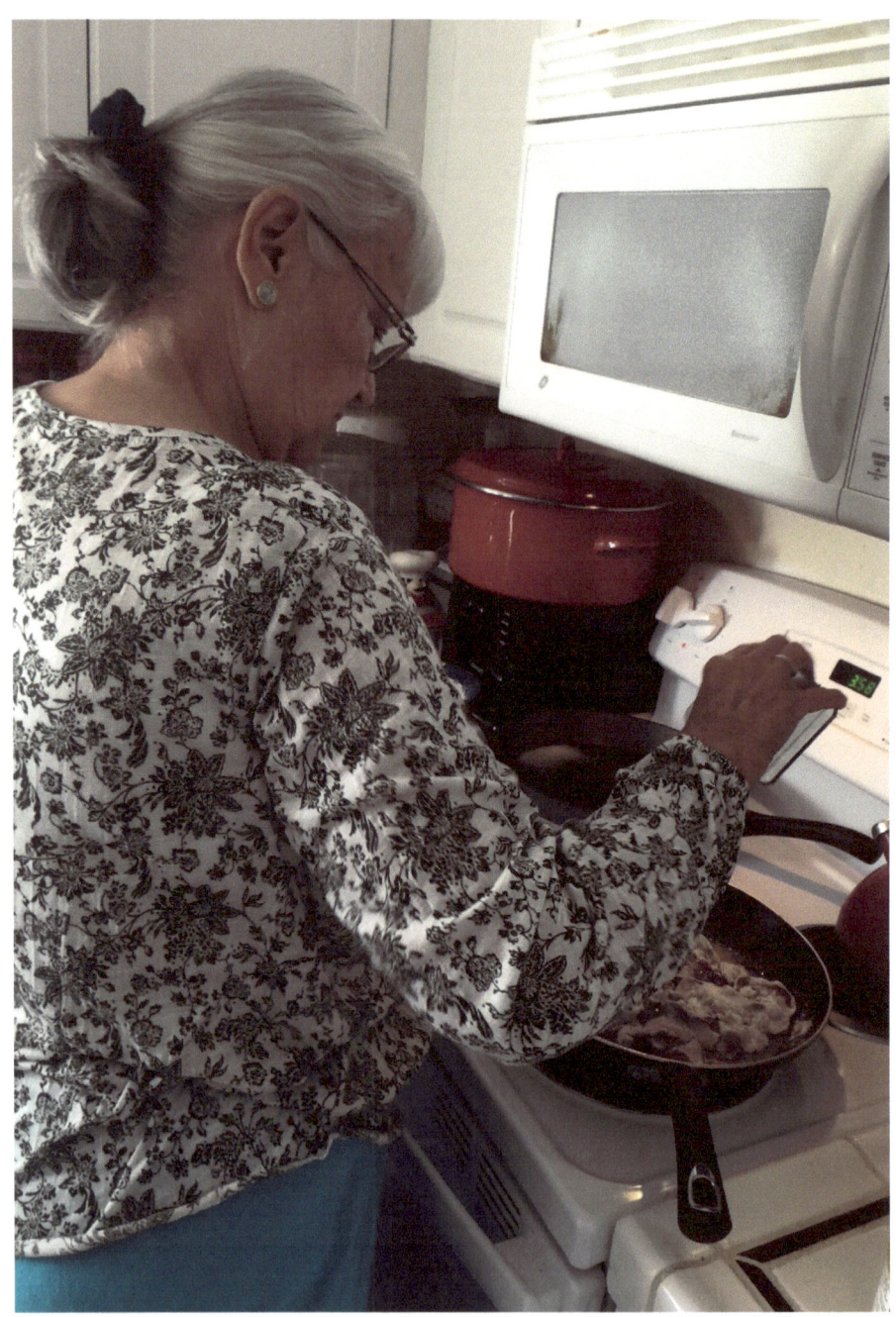

Photo by Dan Tolva

Colleen, wearing turquoise pants, fries up a disgusting batch of chicken livers.

... Doing in a nice girl like you?

looks, and she does, by the way, she still has the pain with which to wrestle.

On the positive side, she actually seems to have grown an inch because the new knee straightened and lengthened her left leg.

Many people remarked about how she seems to have lost weight, and according to the scale, she has lost a few pounds. That tickles her pink but we both agree that getting a new knee doesn't justify this kind of weight loss program.

Nights are still rough. Even with just a couple of pill breaks, It's hard to get back to sleep. That leaves us a bit groggy for the next day.

Colleen also hasn't been driving very much, first due to the pain, and second due to the fact that the oxycodone leaves her woozy to the point she shouldn't be operating heavy machinery.

One thing seems back to normal though: Garage sales.

The other day, while running a few errands, Kasey and Colleen decided to stop in at a garage sale. Like a fool I gave Colleen my last five dollar bill, and she used it to get a turquoise-colored top and slacks.

She put them on later, and I swear it made her look like a Florida senior citizen waiting to croak. That turquoise was awfully popular in the 1950s. I told Colleen, if we put a set of tailfins on her she would look like a 1957 De Soto. But she insists the outfit is very comfortable.

We had planned on going to church today, but partly because we were up in the middle of the night taking pills and administering ice packs, and partly because the knee was still smarting, we had to stay home again. Fortunately, a couple of Priesthood holders brought the sacrament to our home so we could partake of the water and the bread in remembrance of our Savior.

I'm still the chief cook and bottle washer, though she did make herself toast and eggs for breakfast the other day. But she still hasn't washed a dish, which, as recorded earlier in these posts, keeps her on our pampered list. But I really don't mind.

We have physical therapy again Monday, but Karla won't be available to take us, and neither will Kasey, who has to work. Colleen just might have to drive us up there herself. But we will see.

For now we're just going to enjoy a nice quiet Sabbath day. We're having leftover meatloaf and baked potatoes, but Colleen decided to fix herself some chicken livers. Yuck! She's welcome to them.

Stove-top Huffing About My (Hazardous) Cooking Skills

Sept. 26, 2017

Colleen update: Well, actually this is as much a Danial update as it is about our Plucky Lass. Oh, she's plugging along, exercising, taking her pills, walking as far as the mailbox, and being disgustingly cheerful about the whole process.

I, on the other hand, have had a few moments of surliness about me, brought on by cabin fever. Especially with the weather this nice, I want to get out and go.

Instead, it's the same ol' same ol'; waiting for the oven timer to go off, waiting for the suds to settle down so I can see the bottom of the sink, waiting for people to eat so I can collect their dishes. In fact, I feel like a regular homemaker.

This gives me a brand new appreciation for the main women in my life, especially my mom (God rest her soul) and Colleen (God rest her soles). They certainly went through a lot to make sure I was well fed, well clothed, and generally fat, happy and sassy.

So now it's my turn to keep care of the household, and I'm muddling along the best I can. I've certainly gotten to know our kitchen a lot better, where everything is, and I'm getting to be able to decode the confusion of our disgustingly messy pantry.

I suppose any conscientious cook will tell you that there is a certain rhythm

... Doing in a nice girl like you?

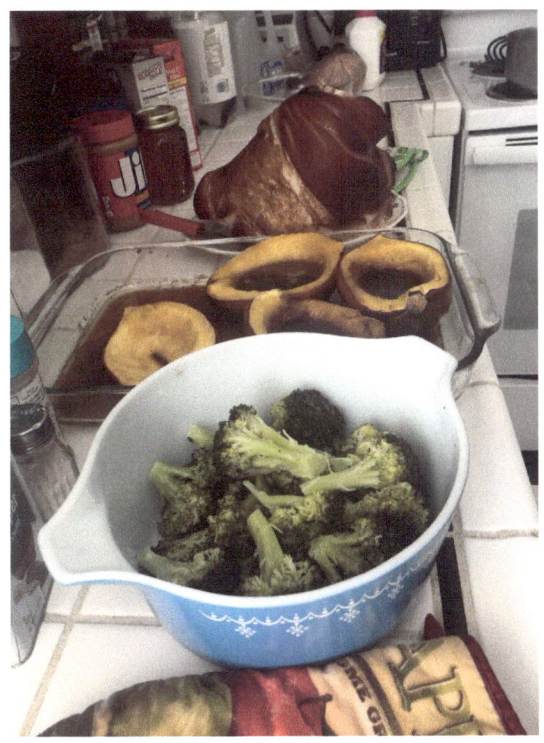

Photo by Dan Tolva

On the menu today: Brocoli, sweet potatoes and ham.

to a well-run kitchen, a symmetry in which everything has a place. It's taking me awhile to discover the rhythm of our kitchen.

Today Colleen and I embarked on our first real grocery-shopping outing since before her knee surgery. We wandered the isles of WinCo filling out a long list. I was pushing a cart, and she was riding one. The rhythm of the kitchen is one thing, but the rhyme or reason behind where WinCo puts groceries befuddled both of us. But we still managed to complete the list in relatively short order.

We managed to get home, fueled by a couple of maple-powered treats. I put all the groceries away while Colleen took a well-deserved Tylenol and laid down. As soon as I got the groceries squared away, I grabbed the two ice packs and iced Colleen up.

Then I got two butternut squash, scooped out the innards, filled the cavities with brown sugar and butter, and plopped the squashes in the oven.

Then I put a big ham in a roaster in the oven alongside the squash.

Twenty minutes or so before the ham and the squash were to come out, I put a couple of bunches of broccoli in the steamer. The broccoli got some salt, pepper, garlic, and butter. That made a wonderful green dish to go with the orange of the squash and the roasty brown of the ham.

Colleen, meanwhile, was on the phone to the Coumadin clinic to try to find out whether she has to keep taking that nasty drug.

Normally, people who get knee replacements need to take Coumadin for a month after the surgery to help avoid blood clots. It has been exactly 30 days since Colleen underwent surgery.

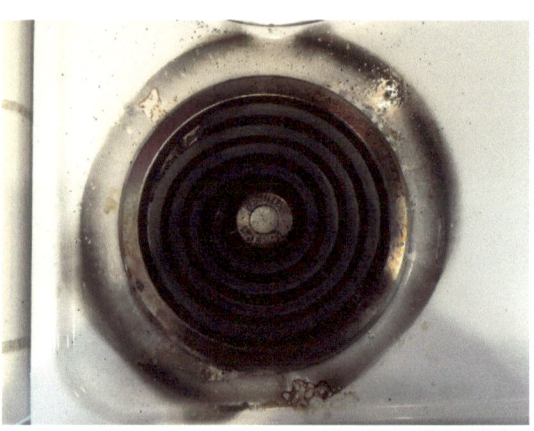

Photo by Dan Tolva

Needed: A little firefighting foam on the range.

Oh, one extraordinary thing did happen to Colleen while I was puttering away in the kitchen. Benny the Cat brought in a little bird, and let it go in Colleen's bedroom, where it flitted about, banging into a mirror and a couple of windows, thereby knocking itself silly and falling under the bed.

We feared the bird was dead. But about 20 minutes later I went out into the kitchen and found the little critter hopping around the windowsill. Colleen caught it, then released into the backyard. We assume it got away OK, but we hope Benny didn't track it down.

Well, it's time to take the food out of the oven and get dinner ready. I'll try to pry Colleen off the phone and with any luck we'll have a nice meal by and by.

...

... The meal was indeed a success. I doctored up the squash by adding a little sour cream to the meat and the brown-sugar mixture, then whipping it into a nice light pudding. Colleen was nice enough to take the innards out of the cook squash skins for me.

But in the interest of full disclosure, I am duty-bound to report that there was a bit of an accident. I was trying to make ham gravy with the burner on high, when a fire erupted around the pan in which I was stirring the liquid.

Even though this was my first kitchen fire, I kept my cool and snuffed out the flames with a lid from another pan.

Of course, the smoke alarms went crazy, the cat freaked out, and we opened all the doors to air out the house. Other than that, dinner was a complete success.

And one last note about Colleen. She passed another milestone of sorts today with her last Coumadin pill. We're both glad to see that regimen end, because that is a nasty, nasty drug. Just one more little step on the road to complete normalcy.

Colleen's Tough Choice

Sept. 27, 2017

Colleen update: I gave our Plucky Lass a couple of choices today: Either let's clean up the pantry, or let's go for a walk somewhere other than to the mailbox.

The first choice was a forlorn hope on my part. After doing most of the cooking the past few weeks, I had grown tired of navigating that really messed up pantry. I was actually afraid that stuff would come tumbling off the shelves and kill me.

So, I offered Colleen the opportunity to help clean up the pantry. All she had to do was sit at the table and tell me where stuff went, and I would've done all the legwork. But no, Colleen protested, her new knee would never take the strain and pain. In fact, her knee probably wouldn't be healed enough to tackle the pantry until late 2021 or early 2022.

Then I offered to go for a walk somewhere other than to the mailbox, which is just 100 yards or so down from our house. I had complained in my last Facebook post but I was going stir crazy because we just haven't had a chance

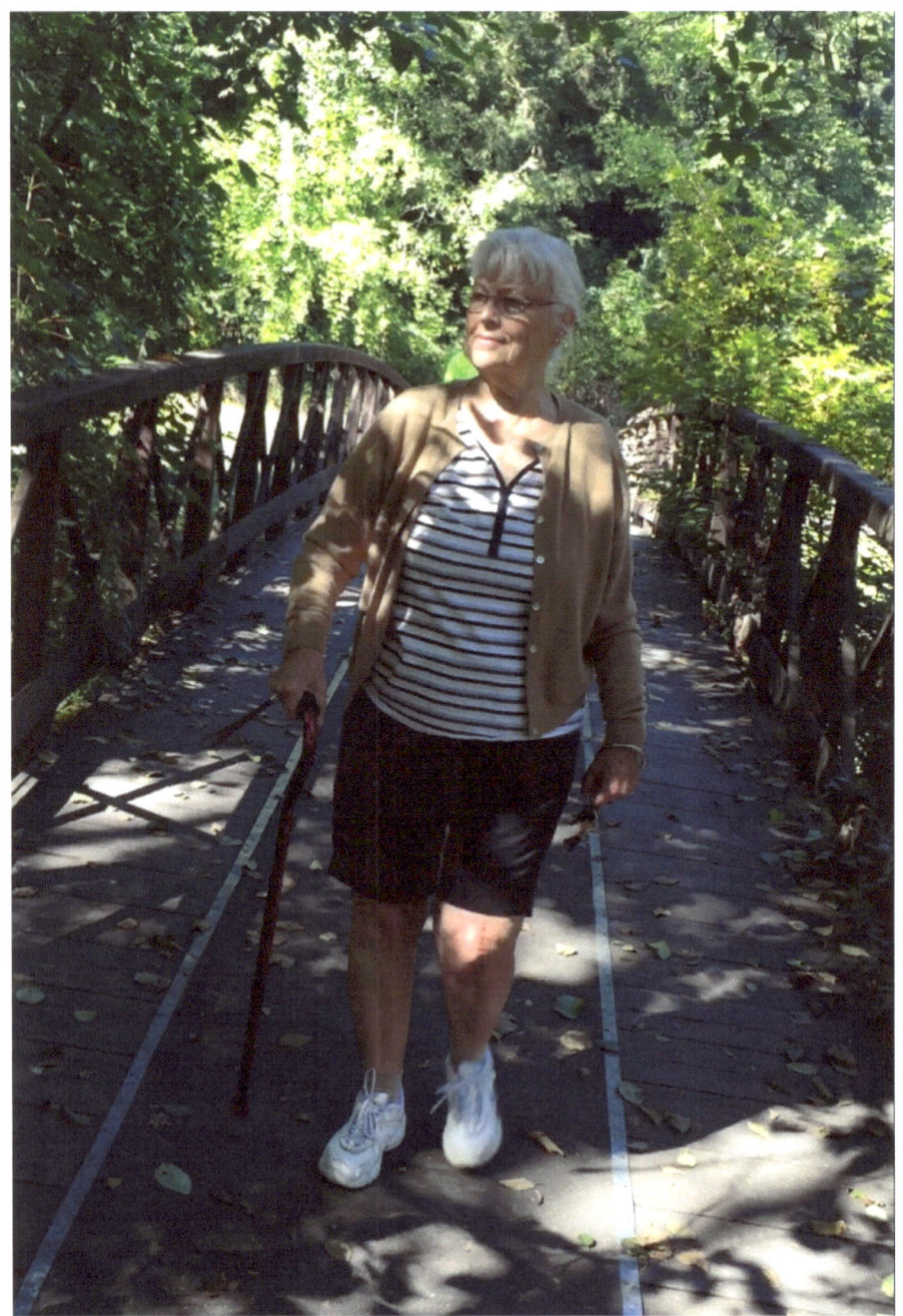

Colleen crosses a foot-bridge on Discovery Trail.

to get out much since Colleen's knee-replacement surgery on Aug. 29.

Colleen's oldest daughter, Kelly Brown Vossenkemper, posted in response that I should take those little walks to the mailbox with my lovely wife to get me out of the house and to get some much-needed exercise. But, I responded, I could still see the cabin that was giving me cabin fever from the mailbox. So what's the point, I asked.

Instead I suggested to Colleen that we go walking along Discovery Trail, which is located in a greenbelt off of Hazel Dell Avenue. It was a perfectly wonderful warm, sunny day for our adventure.

We took a footbridge over a creek, then followed the trail past a pond, and through an archway of green and slightly turning leaves. Dappled light fell on the path, and tiny leaves were skittlering all over the place. It was delightful!

Then Colleen and I drove to her latest round of physical therapy, where she continues to make progress. But the long walk and the therapy combined to give her a lot of pain, so when we got home, I iced her knee down to help ease the swelling and numb the discomfort.

Colleen has her usual bunch of music students this afternoon, and after that, we'll dig into the leftovers of that splendid meal I fixed yesterday. I guess the pantry will have to wait a couple of years or so.

Pantry Project Got My Gloat

Sept. 29, 2017

Colleen update: The bloom is off the rose, our Plucky Lass has lost her magic status as a pampered patient. As of this morning, she's just another lovely wife with a sore knee.

And what brought about this change in status?

This morning, for the first time since before her Aug. 29 knee-replacement surgery, Colleen washed a dish. I had already stated in earlier posts that action would bring an official end to her convalescence.

And the really nifty thing about her doing those dishes is that she did it for me. All because the kitchen was a huge mess because of my latest project, getting our extremely messy pantry into shape.

I started the project two days ago, and have been working pretty much night and day to get it completed. Now the kitchen table and counter are cluttered with pantry debris, awaiting our decision on what to keep and what to toss.

A bout with low blood sugar woke me up this morning at about 4, and because I was awake, and because I had to get up in a little while to remind Colleen of her pill and get grandson Liam off to school, I stayed up and continued my efforts on the pantry. I eventually did go back to sleep.

That's when Colleen, seeing a sink full of dirty dishes and all of the clutter from the pantry on the draining board and kitchen table, took pity on me and

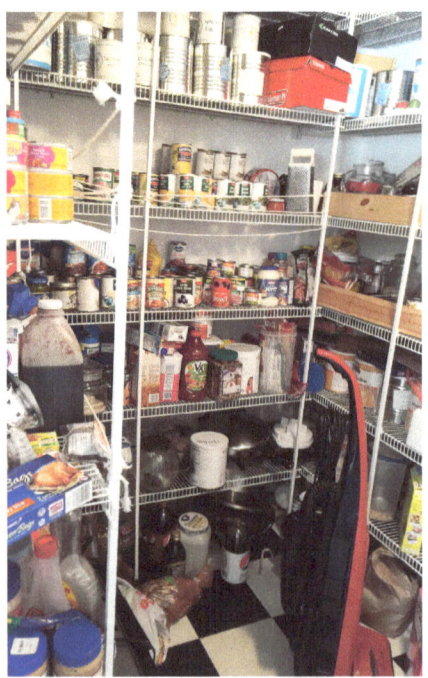
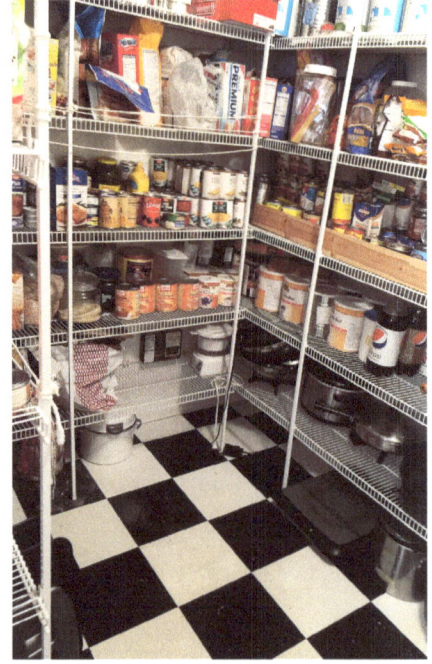

Photos by Dan Tolva

Our pantry before and after clean-up project.

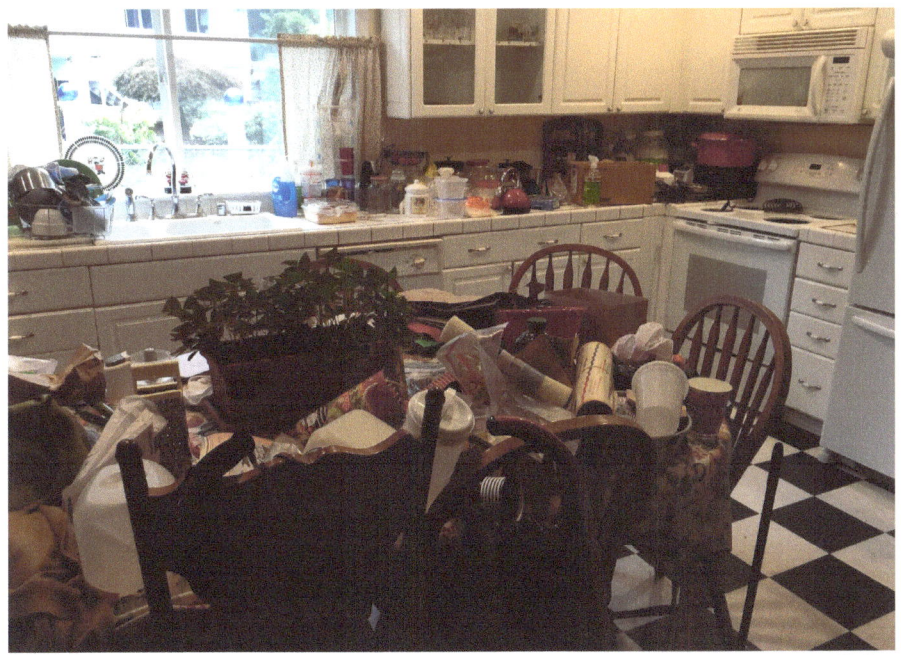
Photo by Dan Tolva

kitchen table covered with pantry stuff during clean-up.

did a slew of dishes from the last day. I had intended on doing them today, so I imagine my relief when I woke up and found that she had done them.

I did get up in time to go with Colleen to physical therapy this morning, where she was put through some new exercises to enhance the improving flexibility of her artificial knee. We'll be adding a few new exercises to the daily routine.

Getting back to the pantry, you can't imagine how pleased I was with myself for just starting the project. In fact, I started this post as a "Danial update" to crow over my glorious actions.

I actually kind of shamed myself into cleaning the pantry because of my last two posts. In them I referred to my messy pantry, and doing so made me feel a little obligated to follow up and do something about the crisis.

Starting at about 10 Wednesday morning, I ventured into the pantry and got to work. I stacked, I unstacked, I stuffed, I unstuffed, I even mopped the floor, and went so far as to launder all of the aprons, napkins, and other assorted pieces of cloth.

Colleen helped sweep and mop the pantry floor. And Liam even took a hand at the broom. But the rest of it was all my sweat and labor.

By the way, Benny the Cat didn't help one bit.

(At the end of this post are three photos showing our cluttered kitchen, the nearly cleaned-up pantry, and Benny the Cat contributing nothing to the effort whatsoever.

So, you ask, am I looking for a reward for my noble effort? I mean, after all, this is akin to Hercules cleaning up the Augean stables. You wouldn't believe the, uh, stuff I found in there.

Am I expecting a reward? You bet your sweet bippy I am. I figure I've already piled up enough brownie points the last month keeping care of Colleen, and this mighty chore can only add to my booty.

I am expecting big things. Especially prime rib. Lots of it.

The Last 'Update'

Oct. 1, 2017

Colleen update: This is likely going to be the last "Colleen update" I'll be writing. This series of posts has been detailing our Plucky Lass's recovery from knee-replacement surgery.

It has been 34 days since Colleen got her new knee, and slowly but surely, she has been growing stronger day by day. Her latest exploit serves as a crowning touch to what was a magnificent effort on her part.

This weekend, she climbed the stairs to our family room for the first time so she could watch our church's semi-annual General Conference from Salt Lake City. Her journey up and down the stairs serves as a symbolic end to this chapter in her life.

Throughout these updates, I have detailed any number of friends and

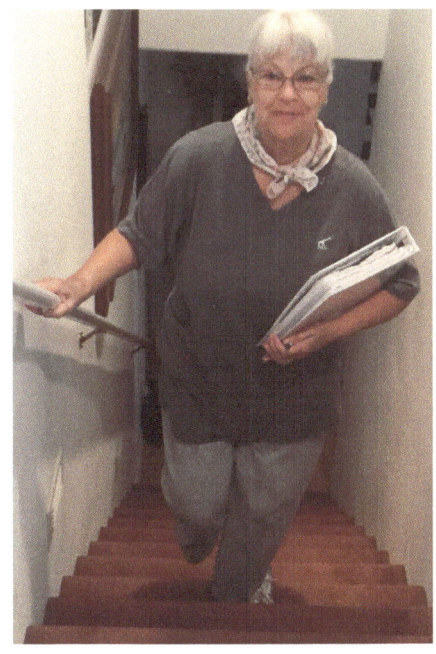

family who reached out to help us cope with Colleen's convalescence. But so far, I have failed to mention perhaps the most important factor in the success of her effort.

Throughout her recovery, and in the rest of her life, Colleen has been bolstered by a deep and abiding faith in Heavenly Father, his son, Jesus Christ, and the Gospel of truth and joy they have brought to the world.

Colleen's strong faith has helped her maintain a positive and cheerful demeanor throughout days and nights often filled with pain. Yet for each tear shed, there have been many more moments of laughter, joy and gratitude for all the helping hands.

Anyone who knows Colleen can testify to her active and boisterous testimony of the Gospel and of the truthfulness of the Church of Jesus Christ of Latter-day Saints.

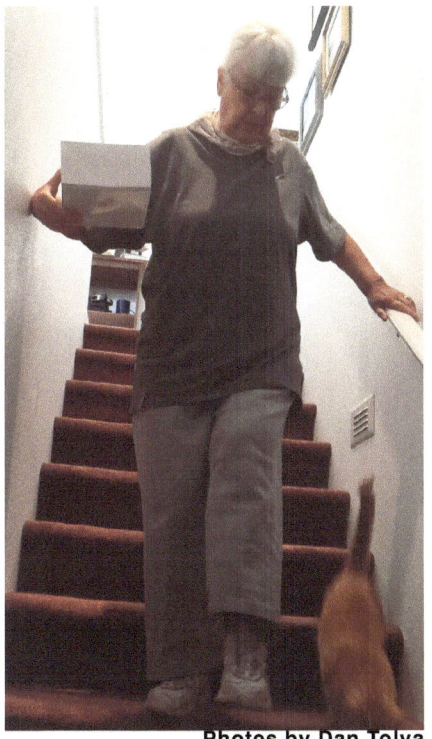

Photos by Dan Tolva

Colleen climbs steps at home for the first time since getting her new knee, and later gets back down, escorted by Benny the Cat.

Supported by her new left knee, Colleen now expects to return to all of her church callings and activities stronger than ever.

She has a Sunday school class to teach, a Ward choir to accompany, any number of families and individuals to contact each month, and of course there is her tireless missionary work.

This doesn't mean the challenge is over. Her caregivers say Colleen can expect pain for several more weeks, which means the medications must continue.

Taking care of my lovely wife all these weeks could've been a real drag.

But she has been such a delight, even when hurting, that it seems like no chore at all.

In fact, this challenge has been so beneficial to our relationship that I'm thinking of whacking her right kneecap with a hammer so we can go through the whole process again.

Not really.

But the experience has been positive, and has given me a new appreciation for family and friends, and especially for the mercy of a tender and just Heavenly Father and his Son.

May God's blessing be upon all of you who have helped and prayed for us in the last five weeks. Your efforts have been wonderful and fruitful.

Springing the Surprise

Oct. 10, 2017

Colleen update: Yes, I know I said I had written the last "Colleen update." What I should have said was, "But wait, there's more!"

OK, so I sound like an infomercial. But there have been a few developments in the life of our Plucky Lass and her new knee, so I thought I'd catch you up.

We have settled into a somewhat normal routine, doing a lot of the usual stuff such as grocery shopping, thrift store hunting, kid hopping, and even

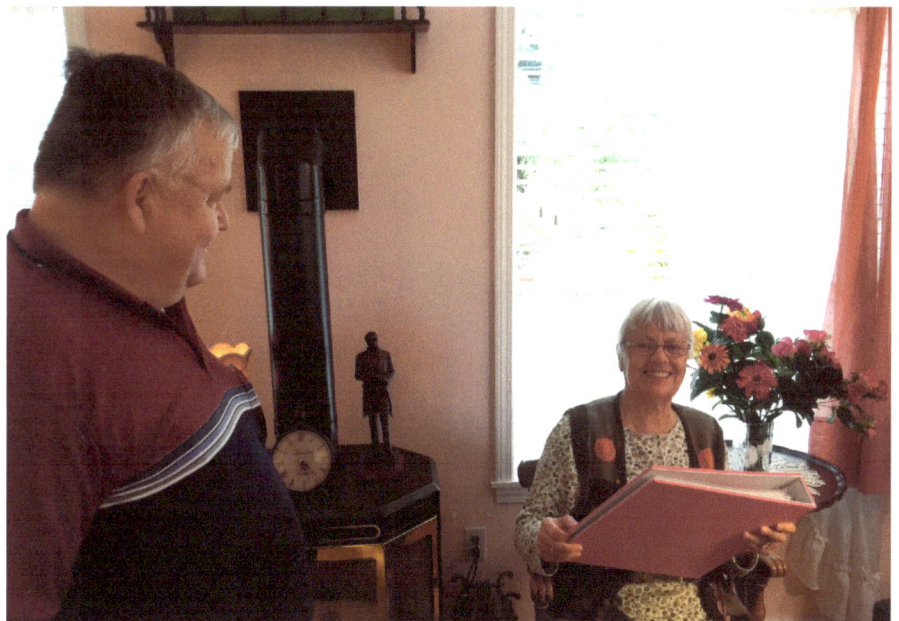

Photo by Kasey Frazier

Dan presents knee-replacement scrapbook to a surprised Collen.

"bomping." Before you get any weird ideas, bomping is our term for piling into the car, snagging a bag of munchies, and wandering around just to see what adventures will come our way.

Colleen actually made it to church Sunday for the first time in five weeks. I, on the other hand, had to stay home largely because of aches and pains suffered while falling from a chair I was occupying in the midst of administering ice to Colleen. Sort of a battlefield injury, you might say.

Nonetheless, we are pretty much back to normal. Unfortunately, the routine also includes wake-up calls at least twice a night for pain pills or ice packs. Our medical caregivers tell us the pain is likely to linger for at least two or three more weeks, and that there could be some discomfort for months. However, Colleen considers the new knee a godsend. She is walking so much more normal now, "not like a penguin," as one of her young music students observed. She

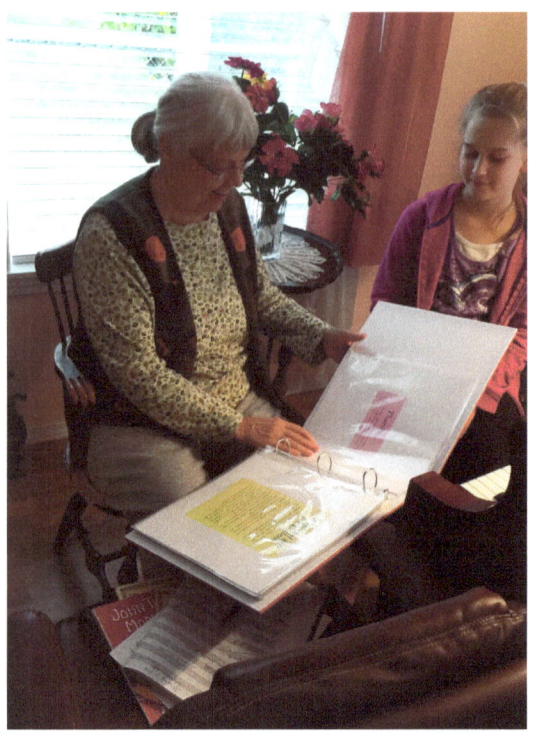

Photo by Kasey Frazier

Piano student Charlotte Dunning gets a kick out of Colleen's new scrapbook.

has remained chipper and cheerful as always.

In fact she's been such a good sport about all of this I thought it would be nice to give her a little present to show my appreciation and admiration for her wonderful spirit. So I devised a scrapbook made up of all of our Facebook posts concerning her knee-replacement surgery, along with many of the photos accompanying those articles.

I found out that scrapbook pages are usually 12-by-12 inches, so I made up a suitable document in the publishing software QuarkXpresss, compiled all of the Facebook posts, and put together 47 pages of material. I also added extra pages so Colleen could paste in a few of her own artifacts. After I had finished compiling the scrapbook in Quark, I converted the whole thing into a PDF file so it could send to the printer.

My co-conspirator in all of this was Kasey, my younger stepdaughter. She drove me to Craft Warehouse and Office Depot, helped pick out materials, hid them at her house, and did a real nifty job of copy-editing proofs.

She also picked up the pages at the printer's, assembled the actual scrapbook, and smuggled it over to our house to be presented to her mom. Colleen, meanwhile, knew something was afoot, because she could see the bills online from Craft Warehouse and Office Depot, and Kasey and I were acting pretty darn conspiratorial. When Colleen asked what was going on, I replied, "That's for me to know and you to find out."

Well, on Tuesday she found out. Kasey, on her way home from work, presented Colleen with the completed scrapbook right in the middle of a piano lesson.

I had shut the front door so Colleen wouldn't see Kasey's van driving up, but my eagle eye wife noticed her arrival and yelled at me that Kasey was out front.

"No she isn't," I said, truthfully, for by that time Kasey had sneaked through the open garage and into the laundry room and was showing me the new scrapbook for the first time. I made a quick check of the page numbers, and Kasey inserted a small photo of Colleen's scar in a sleeve on the cover of the album.

Then, singing "happy un-birthday to you," I carried the album into the living room while Kasey snapped pictures with my iPhone camera.

Colleen loved it. But then, Colleen likes any sort of present. I could've presented her with only a bar of unscented soap marked "occupant," and she would've been as happy as a clam in wet sand.

At any rate, the conspiracy came to a successful conclusion. Thank you, Kasey, for all of your wonderful work. And thank the rest of you for all of your prayers and good wishes.

Hmmmmmm. Now where have I heard that before?

More Positive News

Oct. 11, 2017

Colleen update: Exactly six weeks and a day after her knee-replacement surgery, our Plucky Lass met with one of the surgeons involved in the operation. Physician's assistant Joe Mathias had this cold, clinical medical evaluation

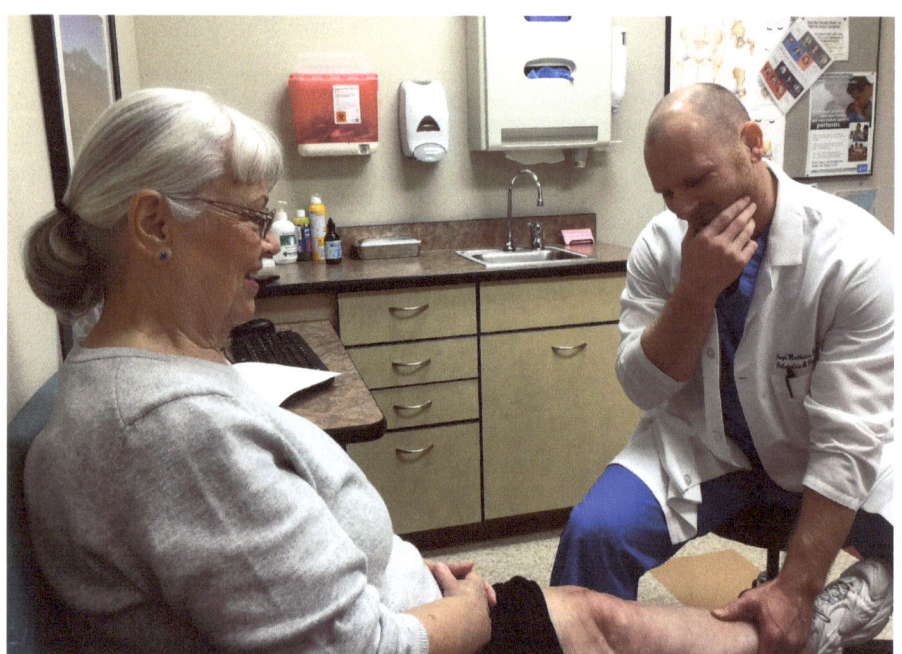

Photo by Dan Tolva

Physician's assistant Joe Mathias ponders Colleen's case ...

of Colleen's progress: "She's really kicking butt."

He poked and prodded the scar, made Colleen hop up and down a little bit, and pronounced her fit as a fiddle, though he did say there would be a lot more pain involved. After all, that is a deep wound the doctors inflicted on her, and it's going to take weeks and weeks to heal completely.

In fact, Joe said, it could be a year before her knee feels back to normal.

We showed the good doctor Colleen's new scrapbook, and he got a big kick out of it. As the surgeon who actually closed the wound, Joe was happy to autograph the picture of the scar used on the scrapbook cover. (See photo below.)

Colleen has to meet with the lead surgeon for her operation, Dr. Cornelius, on Nov. 22. We're going to get him to sign the scar picture as well.

Also today, Colleen had physical therapy for the first time in a week. We

... Doing in a nice girl like you? 47

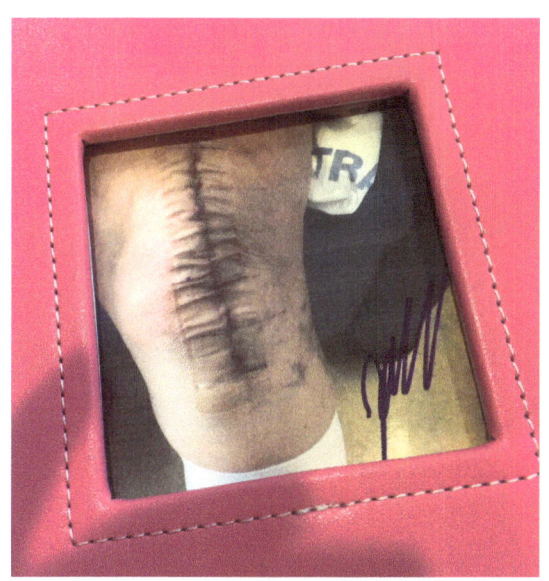

Photo by Dan Tolva

... And autographs the cover of her scrapbook.

were afraid therapist Ali Jakabowski was going to give Colleen a hard time for not doing all of her exercises, but instead, she was impressed with the way Colleen was able to walk, especially up-and-down stairs, and for the strength she is exhibiting in her left leg. Jakabowski said she couldn't even tell Colleen had undergone knee replacement. But that doesn't mean there's not a lot more work to do.

Colleen has another three weeks of physical therapy to go. She's hoping to join a health club so she can keep her new knee limber using the exercise machines.

And everybody loves Colleen's new scrapbook. It's generally agreed that her present will go far in hastening her recovery.

The scrapbook stands at 53 pages today, but it's going to grow as I keep adding Facebook posts. Who knows? Maybe it will have a Volume Two some day.

The Gory Truth

Oct. 12, 2017

Colleen update: For a little change of pace, I thought maybe we could go back to the beginning of this process and give you an idea of what Colleen went through in her Aug. 29 knee-replacement surgery. So I went to YouTube and found a video of a knee being replaced. It's pretty graphic.

In fact, the scene reminded me a lot more of a machine shop than an operating room. The doctors have jigs, hammers, chisels, and drills, not to mention the metal and plastic mechanism of the new artificial knee itself.

There's a lot of hammering. And driving of screws. And as you see, if you have the intestinal fortitude to watch, it's kind of a gory process.

(The next video on YouTube's list was entitled "Knee Replacement Rehab: Top Five Mistakes People Make." I wouldn't dwell on that one if I were you.)

So after looking at all this, it's pretty amazing to me that Colleen has come through this as well as she has, especially with such a wonderful, beautiful, chipper attitude.

And there are a couple of pluses, from her standpoint. First, she got a really neat scrapbook out of the process. Second, she has a whole new round of medical problems to talk about with her friends, family, and whoever else will listen. Even if she stays perfectly healthy from here on, she has an almost infinite supply of new material.

Oh well, that's Colleen, and that's one of the reasons we love her so.

To see the rather graphic video, visit: https://www.youtube.com/watch?v=bGOspdD25Dw.

If you dare.

The Problem With Normal

Oct. 19, 2017

Colleen update: this is getting a little monotonous. After all, how many ways can I say things are getting back to normal and still keep these posts interesting.

Let's face it, normal is boring. Normal doesn't stretch you. Normal does little to excite the senses.

Yet the older we get, the more we appreciate normal. And that's why it's

... Doing in a nice girl like you?

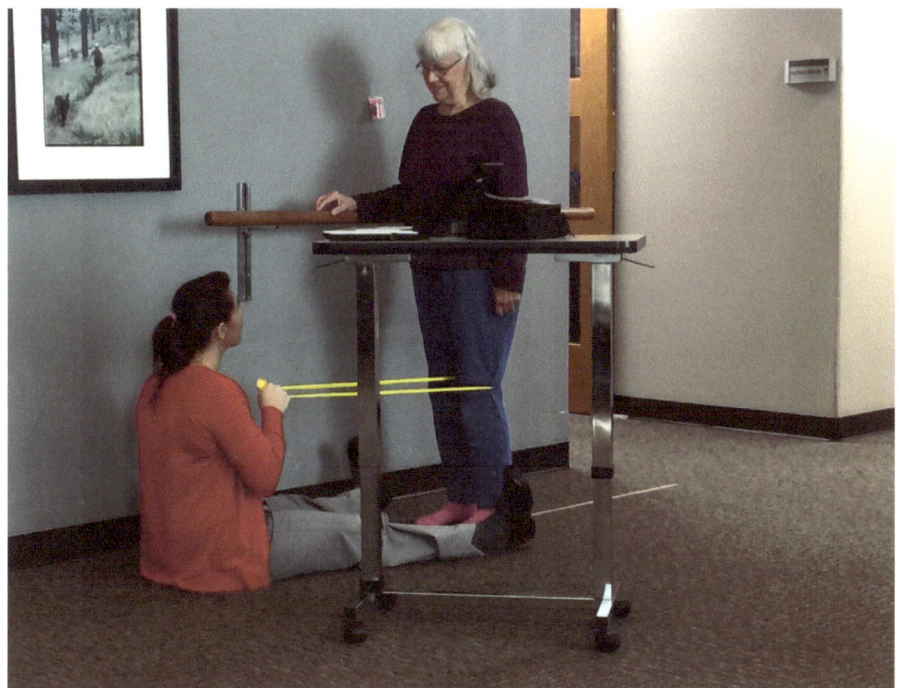

Photo by Dan Tolva

Physical therapist Ali Jakabowski uses elastic band to help Colleen strengthen her new knee and its surrounding muscles.

so neat to see our Plucky Lass assuming many more of her customary ways.

Despite walking around on a new knee, she rarely uses her cane. This is OK, according to her physical therapist, as long as she doesn't overdo it.

We're getting back to our normal schedule in the mornings, usually starting with a phone call from Colleen's oldest daughter, Kelly, prayers, then showers, then breakfast, then kitchen cleanup, then going out into the world to see what adventures await us.

Colleen has long since resumed teaching her full complement of students, and is planning a music workshop for Friday night, and a full recital for Friday, Nov. 10, in the Fries Auditorium at the state School for the Blind.

She's already preparing for Halloween by buying up goodies for trick-or-treaters, an activity she dearly loves to host. Me, I'm not that enthused by a bunch of little sugar-sucking organisms clamoring at our door for stuff that really isn't good for them. I know I'm a bit of a wet blanket, but I never really liked Halloween, even as a kid. But Colleen does, and she actually acts like a kid on the big night, having as much fun as our petite petitioners.

Colleen is still in a lot of pain, especially at night, and this is likely to continue for weeks if not months according to our medical providers. Thank goodness for ice packs, which we use several times a day to help relieve the pain, the heat, and the swelling.

Part of the pain problem is that Colleen has completely weaned herself off the potent anti-pain medication oxycodone. Now she just takes Tylenol four times each 24 hours.

We still have physical therapy for a few more weeks, and one more meeting with the surgeon who performed the knee replacement, Dr. Cornelius. I suppose at that point will be able to say things are completely back to normal. But there are still a few lasting changes in our lives because of this odyssey.

One, I seem to be doing a lot more dishes. I don't like that. But I guess that's a small price to pay for all the prime rib Colleen owes me because I've been such a wonderful person during this time of trial.

(Colleen just heard me dictate that, and made a disparaging sound with her mouth.)

I've also embarked on a couple of new projects related to Colleen's scrapbook. I've completed a smaller pamphlet version of the scrapbook, which I hope to sell to various joint-replacement centers around the country to help reassure those contemplating the surgery that the process can be made easier, especially when you have help from friends and family.

I'm also working on a video using the photos and videos we've posted on Facebook over the last few weeks. That's going a little slower, especially because I don't have any decent audio. I might have to read the transcript of the scrapbook and supply that audio myself.

Family and friends still are offering encouragement and help, for which we remain extremely grateful.

Winding Down, Probably

Oct. 24, 2017

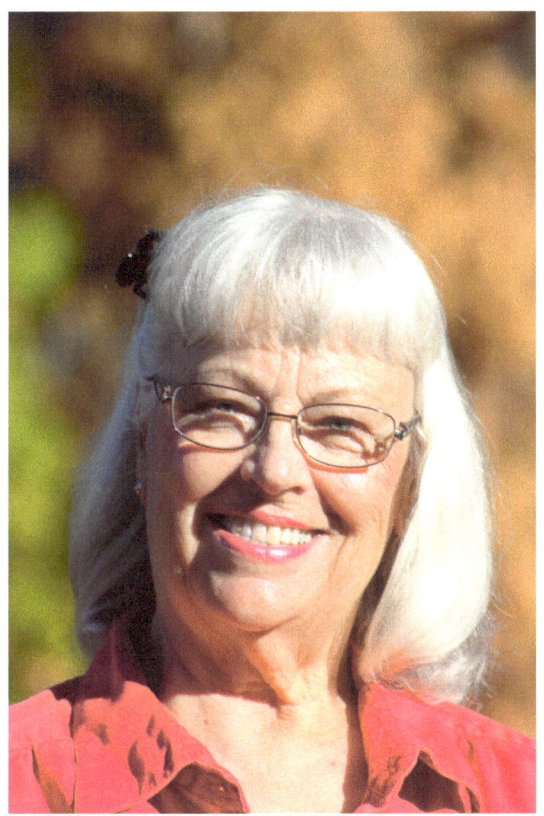

Photo by Dan Tolva

Colleen enjoys a sunny fall day.

Colleen update: Honest, we are closing in on the last of our Facebook updates concerning Colleen and her new knee.

She only has two more physical therapy sessions left, she has weaned herself from the powerful drug oxycodone, and she's walking around usually without the use of her cane.

And she's looking good doing so. Her left knee, which used to be bone on bone and caused her to walk like a penguin before her Aug. 29 knee-replacement surgery, is straight as a board. She's actually gained a quarter inch in height, which she won't let you forget.

To replace regular physical therapy, Colleen has joined a local fitness club to exercise the new knee twice a week or so.

From my standpoint, and we know this whole exercise was all about me,

I've taken all of the prescription alarms off of my iPhone. When we started this process, I had 13 various alarms for assorted drugs throughout the 24-hour day.

But now, Colleen is taking only Tylenol as needed. We are using ice packs a few times a day to fight the swelling and reduce the pain.

Last night, Colleen actually got her own ice packs out of the freezer rather than wake me up. Her motivation was elevated and correct, because anything she can do to ease my considerable burden in taking care of her is a good thing.

We took a drive out towards Ridgefield this sunny beautiful afternoon, and managed to snap a few photos of the fall foliage. We also took the opportunity to record a new photo of Colleen, using our fall colors as a backdrop.

As you can see by the photo below, the expedition was a great success. Doesn't she look cute?

We also used her new photo as part of the printed program for her Nov. 10 recital, to be held at the Fries Auditorium at the state School for the Blind, featuring her piano and violin students.

In three weeks or so, Colleen will meet with Dr. Cornelius, who performed her knee-replacement surgery. We expect his report to be positive, and this event likely will wrap up the series of updates concerning Colleen and her surgery. This should also complete the entries in the scrapbook I made for her, and from which we are developing a book, pamphlet, and video versions.

But, knowing Colleen, there's a good chance we will have plenty of newsworthy events to write about in the next few weeks. After all, Halloween is coming up, and she's promised to go out that night dressed as a healthy person.

A Trip Up the Gorge

Oct. 25, 2017

Colleen update: Well, Colleen's old knee may be gone, but her wanderlust is not.

Our Plucky Lass and I decided to take a drive up to Camas-Washougal to

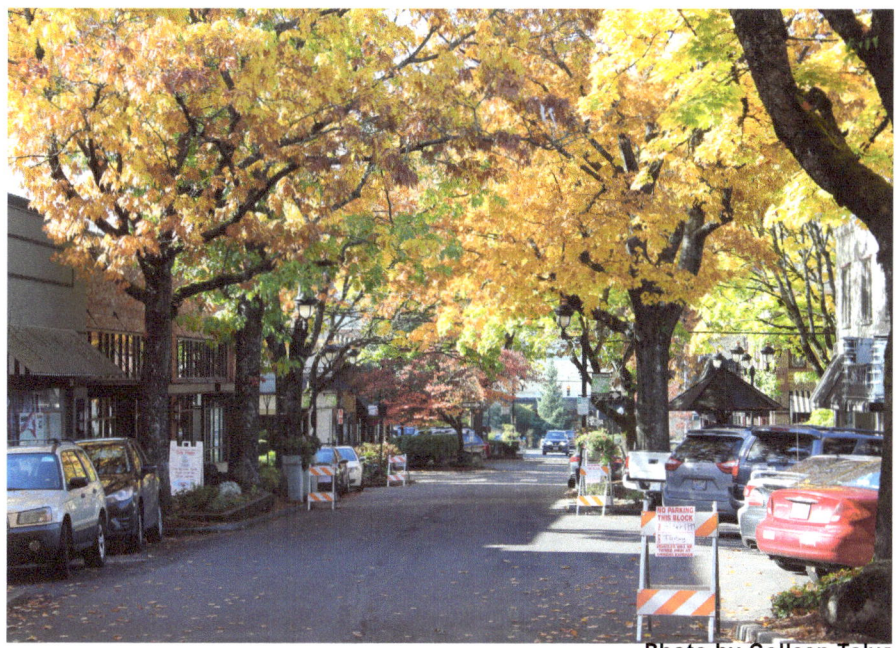

Photo by Colleen Tolva

Downtown Camas in all of its fall splendor.

capture a little fall color on film. But after we got Camas and took a couple of photos, we decided to drive on a little further up the river to the Cape Horn overlook to try to get some more pictures of fall color over the Columbia Gorge.

After a few photos there, we decided to go up to Skamania Lodge for a bowl of soup. That's where the wanderlust ran out, so we turned around, took the Bridge of the Gods over to the Oregon side of the Columbia, and came back home via I-84 and I-205.

On the way, we passed Multnomah Falls and had a chance to look at the damage done by last month's Eagle Creek Fire. The burned-over areas were noticeable, but the damage wasn't as severe as we had feared. There were still plenty of green and gold trees to enjoy.

The whole venture couldn't of taken more than three hours, but that was plenty of time to have fun while not taxing Colleen's new knee too much. Nonetheless, she was still pretty sore by the time we got home.

What's a joint like this ...

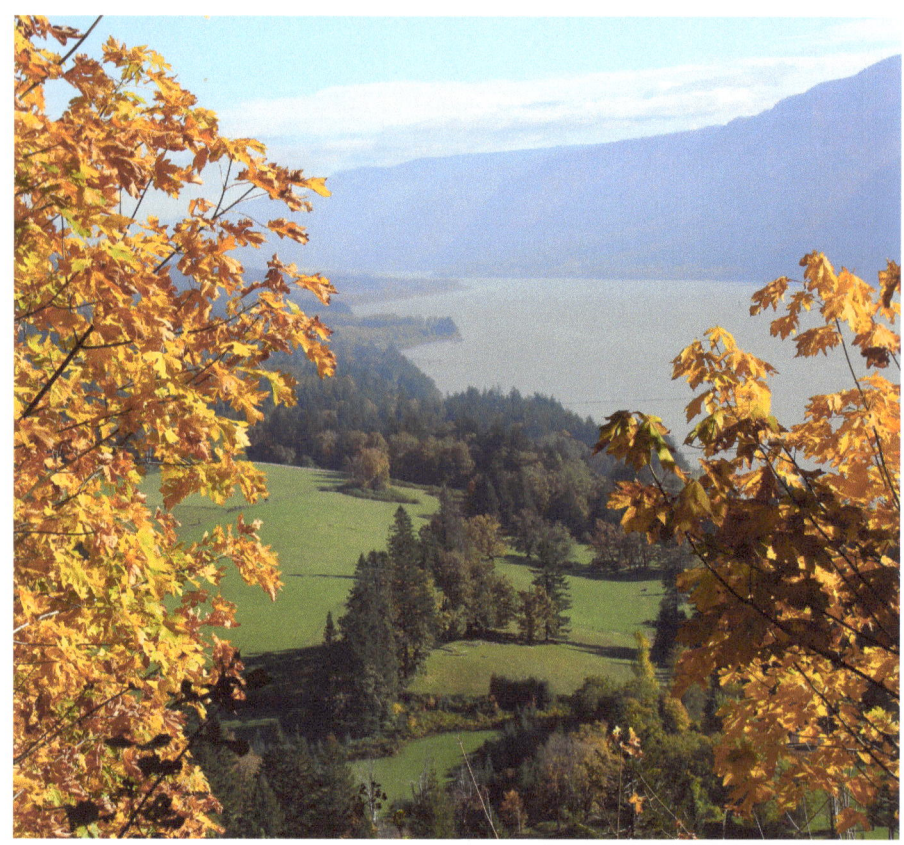

Photo by Dan Tolva

The Columbia Gorge sparkes on a sunny fall day.

    We had a lot of fun, as we usually do on these little day trips around the area. With any luck, our range will increase as Colleen's new knee and its surrounding muscles get tougher over the next few weeks.

Sadness and a Little Joy

Nov. 1, 2017

    Colleen update: With next Friday being the last date for our Plucky Lass's physical therapy, we needed another source of regular exercise.

    So, Colleen joined Planet Fitness to take advantage of the club's many

... Doing in a nice girl like you?

exercise machines. She has been going to the place three times a week, sometimes with her granddaughter, Jessie, who is also a member and who introduced her to the club.

An accompanying photo shows one of the machines Colleen is using. I declined to record her using a machine that required her to move her knees in and out. The last thing I wanted was a picture of my 74-year-old wife looking like she was storing in a Suzanne Somers Thigh Master commercial.

Sadly, Colleen has weightier matters on your mind at the moment. Her sister, Bonnie Gerdes, is suffering from advanced COPD, And the prognosis doesn't look good. Bonnie is being moved into a nursing home today.

Colleen's half-sister and her husband, Carol and Lance, offered to pay Collen's plane fare back to Wisconsin to see Bonnie. But, despite her excellent progress in recovering from her Oct. 29 knee replacement surgery, Colleen is no shape to spend hours on a plane. She is understandably upset that she's not going to be able to see her sister anytime soon, but we're holding out hope that she'll be able to visit her later, perhaps after Thanksgiving.

Colleen has been having fun this week, however. As it turns out, the Halloween season is one of her favorite times of year. She loves orange lights, trick-or-treaters, and the excuse to wear pumpkin-shaped earrings.

This Halloween she greeted dozens of trick-or-treaters late into the evening, requiring each recipient of candy to do some sort of trick. The trick could be as easy as singing a song, or hopping on one foot.

Despite the really nice weather, we got a lot fewer trick-or-treaters than normal this year. That means we have a lot of candy left over, which will delight grandson Liam to no end.

We have been enjoying a glorious fall season of bright, mild days. The foliage is more vivid and beautiful than in years past, it seems. Colleen has been busy photographing the scenic splendor.

After Friday's last physical therapy session, the next significant date is Nov. 22, when Colleen has her final meeting with the surgeon who gave her the new

What's a joint like this ...

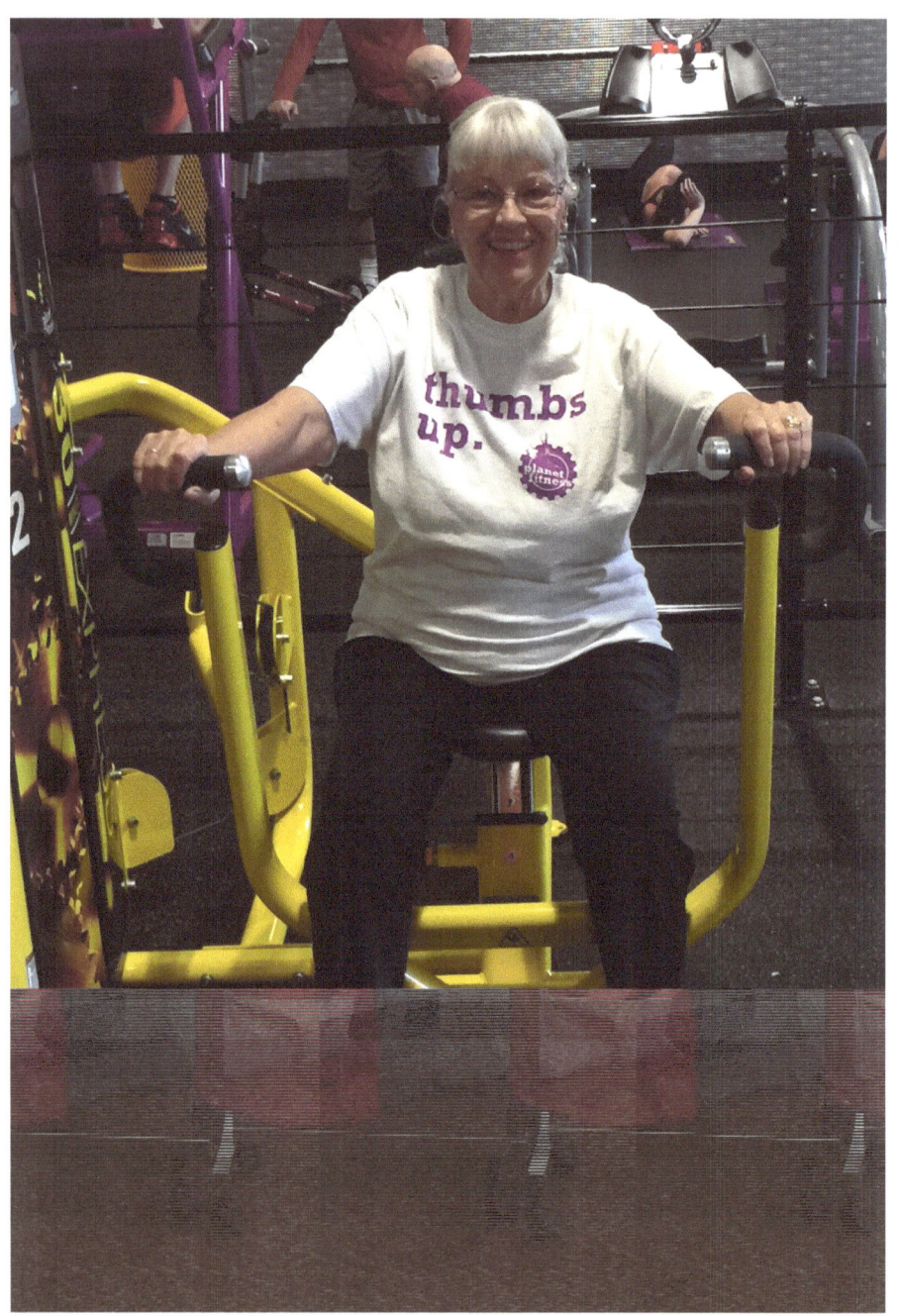

Photo by Dan Tolva

Colleen makes a great poster girl while working out at Planet Express.

knee, Dr. Cornelius. I imagine his report will be the basis for our final "Colleen update" posts.

Until then, we will continue to update Colleen's knee-replacement scrapbook, and continue adding material from that scrapbook to a pamphlet and book detailing this months-long process.

We hope to publish these materials to provide information and inspiration for others contemplating joint-replacement surgery.

Happy Birthday to Me

Nov. 3, 2017

Colleen update: Another milestone for our plucky last came today with her last formal physical therapy session.

Since her Aug. 29 knee-replacement surgery, Colleen has been attending regular physical therapy sessions at the Salmon Creek Clinic. For most of those sections, her therapist was Alexandria "Ali" Jakabowski, who on the outside looks like a kind enough lady but on the inside has the heart and temperament of a Marine drill sergeant.

All along, Ali made no bones about her outlook. She was the boss, and it was up to Colleen to follow orders or else. Fortunately, we never found out what the "or else" entailed. Colleen made it through her last session with flying colors.

The next date of significance for Colleen is Nov. 22, when she is scheduled to have her last meeting with Dr. Cornelius, the surgeon who gave her the new knee. That should wrap up the formal medical process, though healing will continue for weeks and months, as well as a certain level of pain.

But look at everything Colleen has accomplished. She weaned herself off of the powerful opiate oxycodone, she takes Tylenol only rarely now, though she does use ice packs regularly to help curb the pain and swelling in her left leg.

Colleen is doing everything she did before the surgery, and more. She's walking in a much more normal manner than before the surgery, she professes

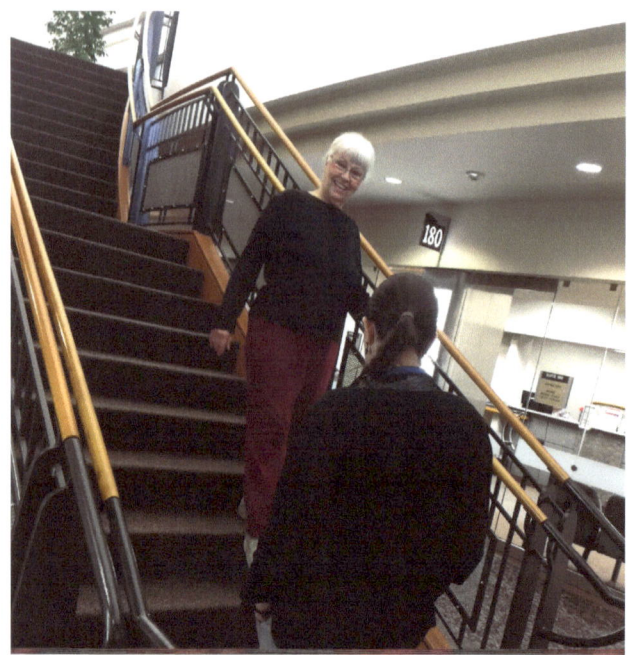

Photo by Dan Tolva

In their final session, physical therapist Ali Jakabowski leads Colleen down a flight of stairs.

to have more energy, and a pesky cough that has bothered her for years seems to have gone away for the most part, knock on wood.

She's back to her full teaching schedule, she has resumed her duties as Sunday school instructor, and she's taking on a new task, accompanying the symphony orchestra she founded back in 1988 on the piano.

For the last couple of days, Colleen has been running around like a chicken with her head cut off getting ready for my birthday. The table is set, presents delivered, and most of our family came over Friday night to share in my main birthday present from Colleen: two big prime rib roasts.

Many's the Facebook post over the last few weeks in which I've expressed my love for this wonderful meat, and I made it clear several times that the reward for taking care of Colleen through all of these trials really needed to be prime rib. Lots of it.

Colleen came through like a champ, with the result that I've spent most of the day preparing the two roasts. Even as I write this, their aroma is invading every corner of the house, and I can hardly wait to tuck in.

I have to quit writing for a little bit now because the family should be

... Doing in a nice girl like you?

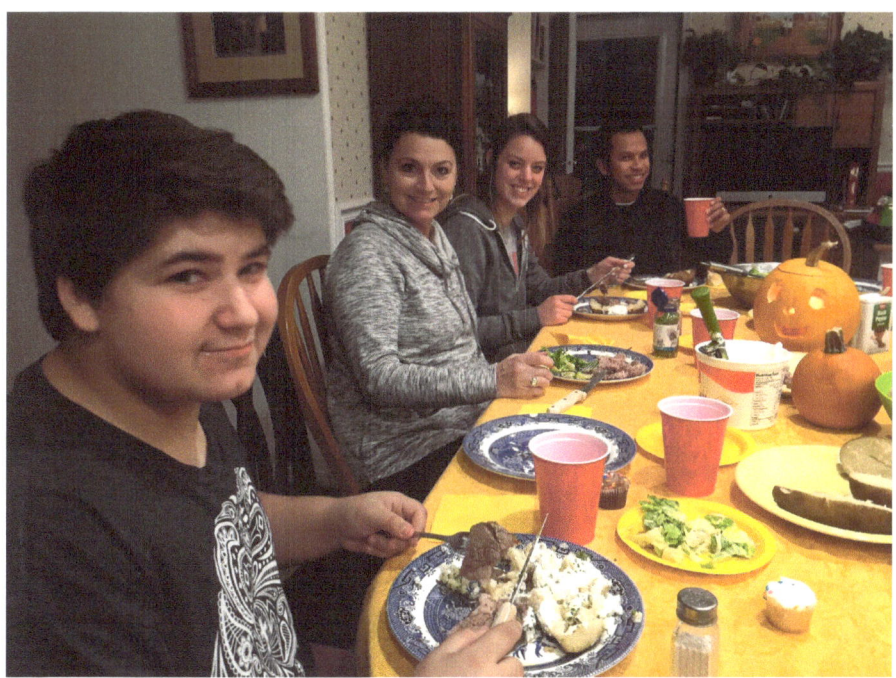

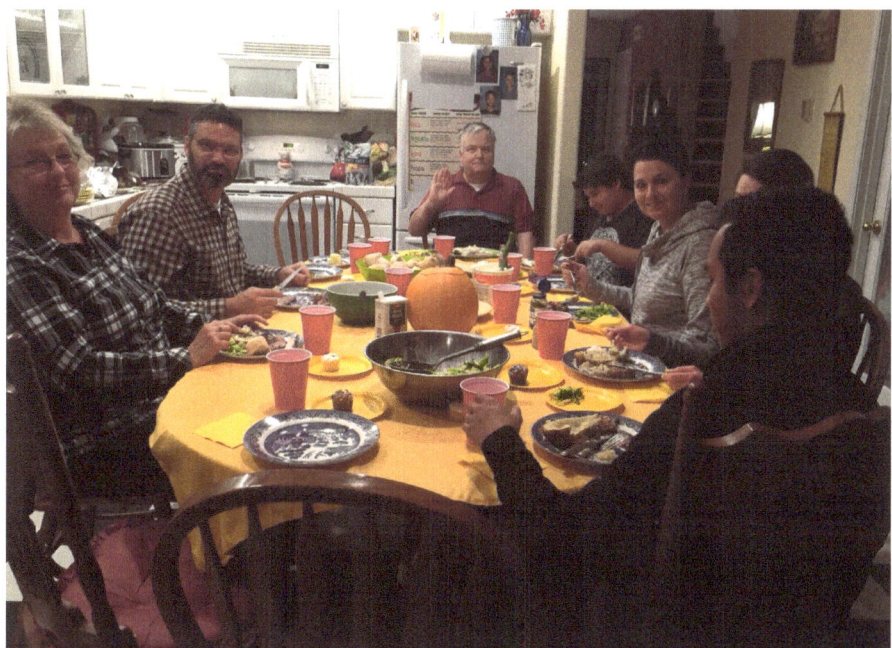

Photos by Dan Tolva

family members join Dan Tolva for a birthday dinner.

arriving pretty soon, and I still have to get the roast out of the oven and prepare au jus gravy to pour over the meat.

Colleen and I put 11 huge potatoes in the oven to bake earlier in the day, and they are now sitting in two crockpots, keeping warm and waiting to be served.

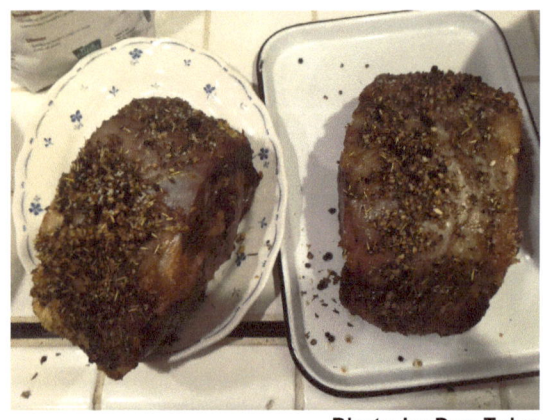

The real star of the evening.

I'll get back to you after dinner, and after the family and I have finished celebrating my 68th birthday. See you in a bit …

… Well I'm back, and Colleen and I couldn't have had a better time.

At about 6 p.m., Colleen's Son, Kevin, and his wife, Karla, arrived. Kevin carved to prime ribs, which had emerged from the oven perfect.

Then came Colleen's oldest daughter, Kelly, and granddaughter Jessica and her husband, Aref. My grandson, Liam, joined us and we all had dinner.

At about 7:30 p.m., Colleen's youngest daughter, Kasey, her husband, Mike, and their three kids, Austin,

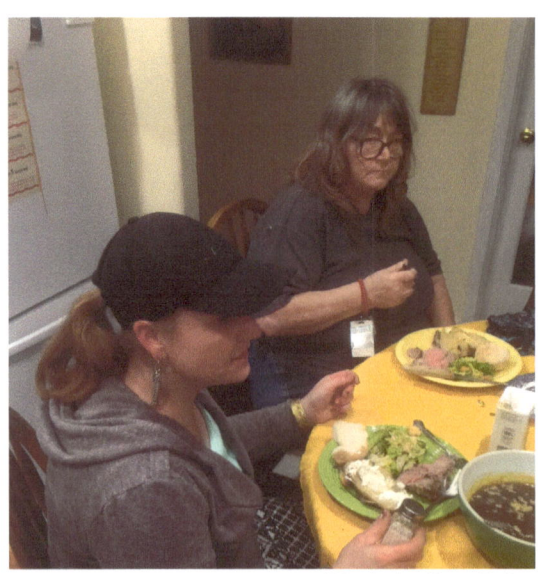

Dan's daughter, Megan, and sister, Valida, enjoy a birthday meal.

Jaden, and Jordan, showed up, and they all chowed down.

Then we adjourned to the living room, where I received all kinds of cards and presents, and we socialized for least a half hour.

Then, wonder of wonders, my younger daughter Megan, showed up with my sister, Valida, in tow. This was a real miracle, because Valida has a lot of trouble getting around, and getting in the car and traveling across the river from St. John's, Oregon, to Hazel Dell was quite an ordeal for her. It had been years since Valida had been over to the house.

Boy, was it wonderful to see her! Like the rest of our guests, she loved the prime rib. I guess this figures, because Valida was actually the one who taught me how to cook the meat.

Eventually, the guests all trickled out, leaving Colleen and I with a wonderfully quiet house and memories of a truly outstanding birthday.

The Surgeon Speaks

Nov. 22, 2017

Colleen update: Today marked a huge milestone in our Plucky Lass's recovery from her Aug. 29 knee-replacement surgery.

Dr. Casey Cornelius, who gave Colleen her shiny new knee, met her for the first time since the surgery and pronounced her fit as a fiddle, though she'll likely suffer some pain for the next several weeks or months.

Dr. Cornelius moved Colleen's left leg around a bit, took a look at the healing but still nasty looking scar, and

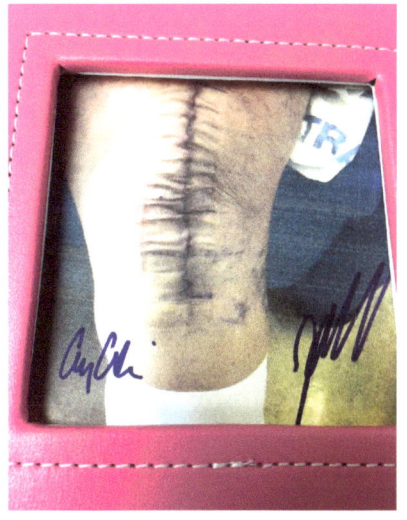

Dr. Cornelius added his signature to the cover of Colleen's scrapbook.

compliment her on her progress. Not only was he impressed with Colleen's care and positive attitude, he really enjoyed the scrapbook chronicling her adventures since the surgery.

The good doctor was also kind enough to autograph the front panel on the scrapbook, with his signature joining that of physician's assistant Joe Mathias, who stitched up the incision.

We told Dr. Cornelius about our plans to turn the scrapbook into a real book aimed at allaying the concerns and fears of those contemplating joint-

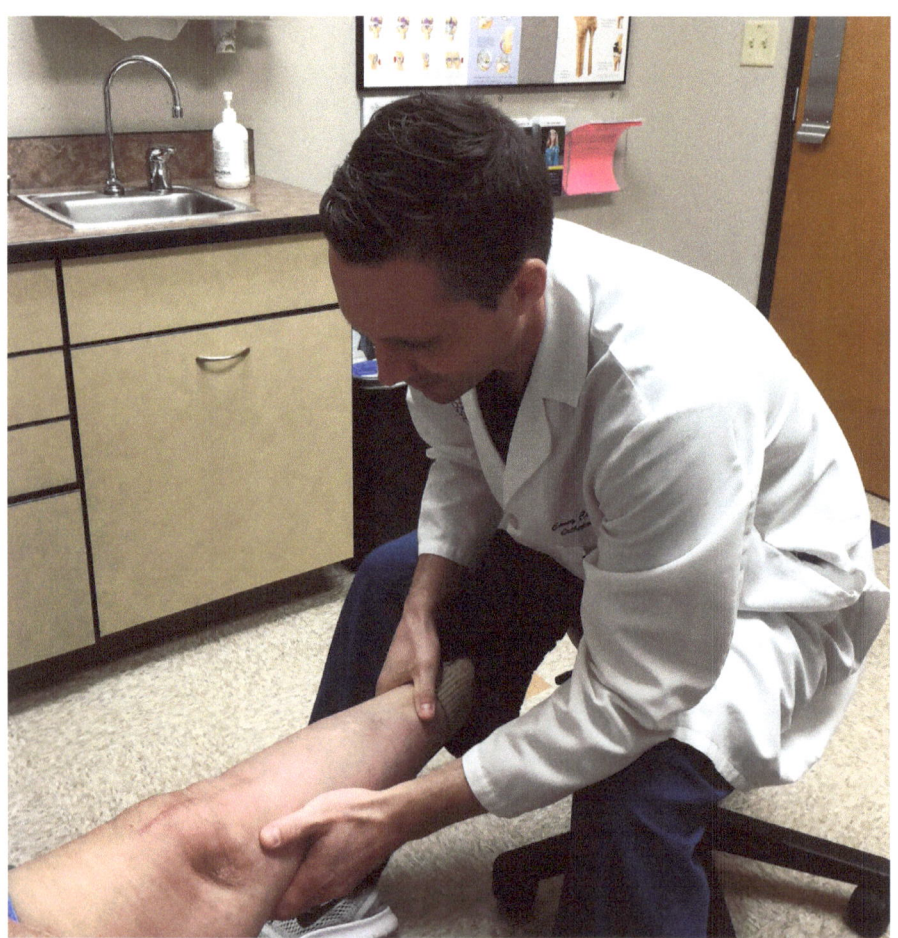

Photo by Dan Tolva

Dr. Casey Corneluis pokes and prods Colleen's knee.

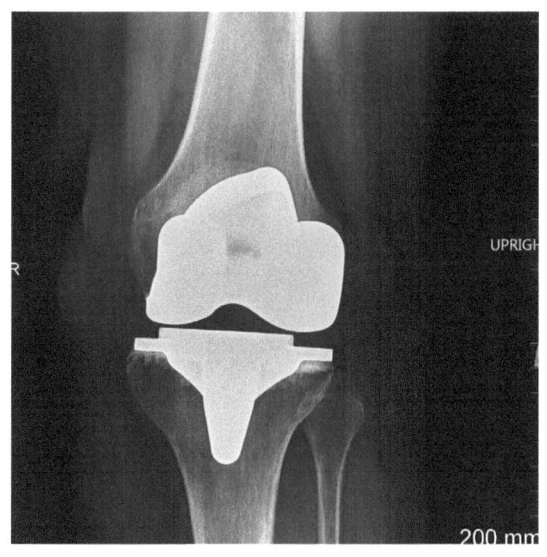

Here's Colleen's new knee.

replacement surgery. Dr. Cornelius speculated that tens of thousands, even hundreds of thousands, of people undergo the procedure in the U.S. each year.

Before meeting with the doctor, X-rays were taken of Colleen's left leg. The Salmon Creek Clinic Image Center provided us with copies of those pictures, along with X-rays taken before the surgery.

I asked Dr. Cornelius if he would write a foreword for our new book, and he said yes. I'll send him a .PDF file of a draft of "What's a Joint Like This Doing in a Nice Girl Like You?" so he can prepare his contribution. His piece, along with some thoughts from Colleen herself, will complete the book.

And the scrapbook will be done, too. It has been a labor of love, appreciated greatly by Colleen and admired by all who have seen it. Now all we need to do is find a publisher.

A Little Stumble

Nov. 30, 2017

Colleen update: Well, our Plucky Lass continues to progress in recovery from knee-replacement surgery, to the point where a big part of the day might go by without her being aware of any discomfort at all.

A few times now she has awakened in the morning with her knee giving her no trouble whatsoever. She is taking much less Tylenol, and using ice packs much less often.

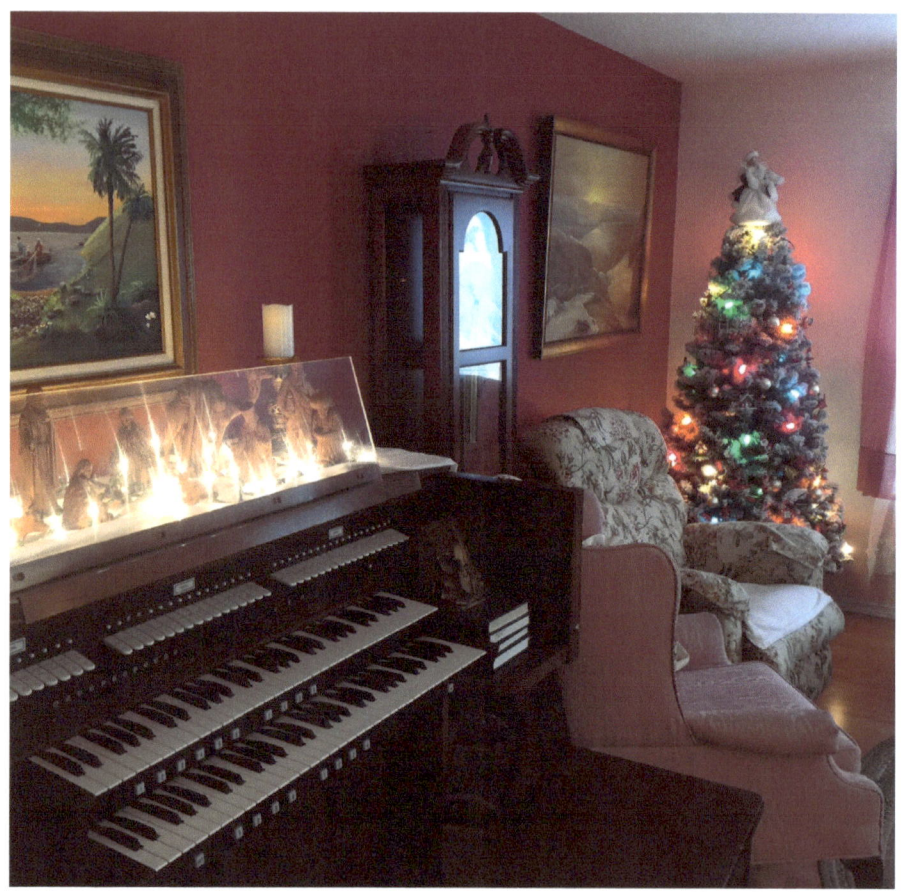

Photo by Dan Tolva

Colleen's organ gets a set of holiday lights.

But that doesn't mean she hasn't had a challenge or two. Take today, for example, when she stumbled while exercising at planet fitness and landed on her new knee.

Although her knee smarted, especially around the area of the incision, the mishap was not a catastrophe. We were careful to ice her up when she got home to combat any swelling. I'm sure she'll have a nasty bruise there for a while. The mishap actually confirms how well she's doing in recovering completely from her Aug. 29 surgery. She is right on schedule according to her medical care givers predicted timetable for the pain to finally go away completely.

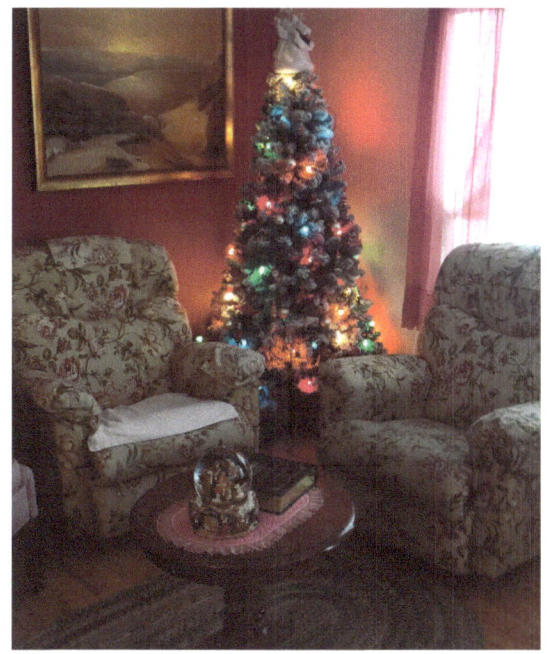

Photo by Dan Tolva

This year's Christmas tree.

Adding to the challenge has been coping with the death of her beloved sister, Bonnie, last Sunday. The funeral was held in Wisconsin Wednesday, but Colleen was unable to attend because of her knee. So she spent hours on the phone with her sisters, brother, and other relatives back in the Midwest, getting reports on how the funeral went.

Relatives also sent photos of the service, which by all accounts went really well. We played a part in the funeral by providing a slide show on Bonnie's life that was projected onto a wall for over two hours as a background to the service.

We were happy and blessed to contribute in a positive fashion, and hope that the slide show will continue to be a valued keepsake for all of those who love Bonnie.

Colleen's three kids, Kevin, Kelly, and Kasey, helped pick up their grieving mom's spirits considerably by sending her a beautiful plant that of course got her all weepy again. As if Colleen didn't have enough to cry about.

Meanwhile, life goes on. Colleen continues to bake the world's best chocolate chip cookies, and continues to eat a good number of them. She is fully back into the swing of things when it comes to cooking, cleaning, her church duties, and teaching music students. And of course there's Christmas to get ready for, and she's all in with that.

I say more power to her.

Back to the Doc

Dec. 4, 2017

Colleen update: That little stumble a few days back turned out to be more trouble than we thought. Our Plucky Lass, while exercising at planet fitness, took a bit of a fall and landed on her new knee.

She didn't land hard, but it was enough to cause a little pain and swelling. She called Dr. Cornelius's office, and they suggested a trip to urgency care and much more use of ice packs.

Colleen decided not to go to urgency care, but we did increase the frequency of icing her leg down. She continued all of her normal activities, and didn't seem to slow down a bit.

Today, we visited Dr. Cornelius again, and Colleen got another X-ray. The doctor examined the knee and declared that all was well, and advised Colleen to stay the course on her road to recovery. We'll return to see him in a couple of months for one more follow-up visit.

After the doctor's visit, Colleen rewarded herself with a yogurt treat and a trip to the gym. But how anyone could regard a trip to the gym as a reward for anything is beyond me.

A Word From Colleen

Dec. 6, 2017

I'm the "Plucky Lass" my sweet husband has been writing about through all these posts and pictures throughout my knee replacement recovery, some of which I asked him not to display.

Oh well, I guess I'm glad he has a mind of his own!

As this wonderful scrapbook came forth and has continued on, it has come to both of our minds that perhaps this story would be useful to others who are anticipating having total knee replacement. It's not sugar coated by any means. But the humor throughout the book should lighten your burden in two ways: first in making the decision to go ahead with your surgery, and second to help you get through the healing process and the intense physical therapy which is so vital to your recovery.

Let's start back at the beginning about a month out from my actual surgery. That's when my care-giver (my sweet husband) and I attended a joint-replacement class at Legacy Salmon Creek Hospital in Hazel Dell, just north of Vancouver, Wash. In a fairly large room was an oversized, rectangular table with many people sitting around (with their caregivers) ready to receive instructions and understanding about what to expect from their upcoming surgery. Nobody smiled, and as I looked around at their faces I could see that they were pretty apprehensive about the whole thing. I also listened carefully to our instructor who was quite pleasant and who herself had experienced more than one knee surgery. I trusted her instructions.

She held up a model knee joint for all of us to see and showed how the titanium joint would perfectly move in our knee. It was an excellent model of the knee. As she continued to speak she sat the model down on the table right in front of my husband.

Danial is legally blind and wanted to really understand what was going on, so he picked up the model and brought it close to his eyes so he could see it better. It was then that the mood changed from solemnity to laughter as the whole model knee just fell apart, hitting the table with a loud thud! Danial looked up and said, " Of course, I'll be the one doing your surgery today!" It was so funny and really "broke the ice," so they say.

On the morning of the surgery, the prep was pleasant and they continually kept a heated plastic gown on me. It really felt wonderful and kept my anxiety down to a minimum. I chose to have a spinal injection rather than be put out with a general anesthetic. (You will be given materials ahead of time to read in

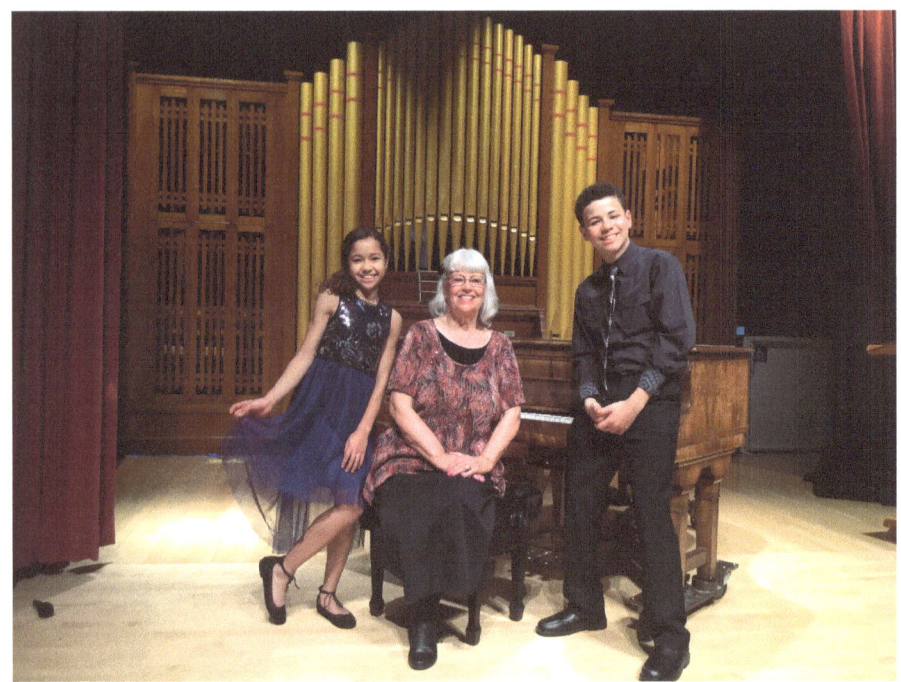

Photo by Kasey Frazier

Colleen poses with two of her music students, granddaughter Jaden, left, and grandson Austin at their fall recital Nov. 8, 2017, at the Washington State School for the Blind's Emil Fries Auditorium.

regards to your choice of anesthesia and other things you'll need to know.)

The surgery went well. Soon I was in my room, and the healing began.

I believed and now know that the caregiver is a very important part of your recovery. I have been truly blessed to have had Danial as my caregiver. As you have read the posts he recorded, you can see that it took quite an effort of patience and kindness on his part not only getting up throughout the night to give me my much-needed pain medicine but to also make sure I did every one of my exercises. If it wouldn't have been for him, chances are I would have backed off when the going got rough!

I hope he receives many choice blessings from heaven. Well, his first one came with the prime rib dinner! That's really all the thanks he's getting! I love him and have to say that service to one another brings you closer together.

One of my favorite scriptures out of The Book of Mormon says, "When you are in the service of your fellow beings you are only in the service of your God."

I must thank my Father in heaven also and his son, Jesus Christ, for watching over me and being there for me when times got rough.

This whole process is amazing to me. The modern technology and the improvement made down through the years in knee replacement (and I'm sure that includes hip-replacement surgery) makes it a definite choice for those suffering with bone on bone. I waited an awfully long time for mine. Even way back in my 30s the doctors wanted to do the surgery, but I held off for 44 years! It was obviously my time to experience this, and, oh my goodness, am I ever grateful I made the choice when I did. As I write this I am 10 weeks out from my surgery, and still experiencing some pain and swelling.

It will take a while for my knee to totally heal. Ice really helps, and Danial still brings it in for me from the freezer and plops it on my knee whenever I need it. I can walk anywhere I want to go. It feels so good. I have a whole new life ahead of me, so look out world, here I come!

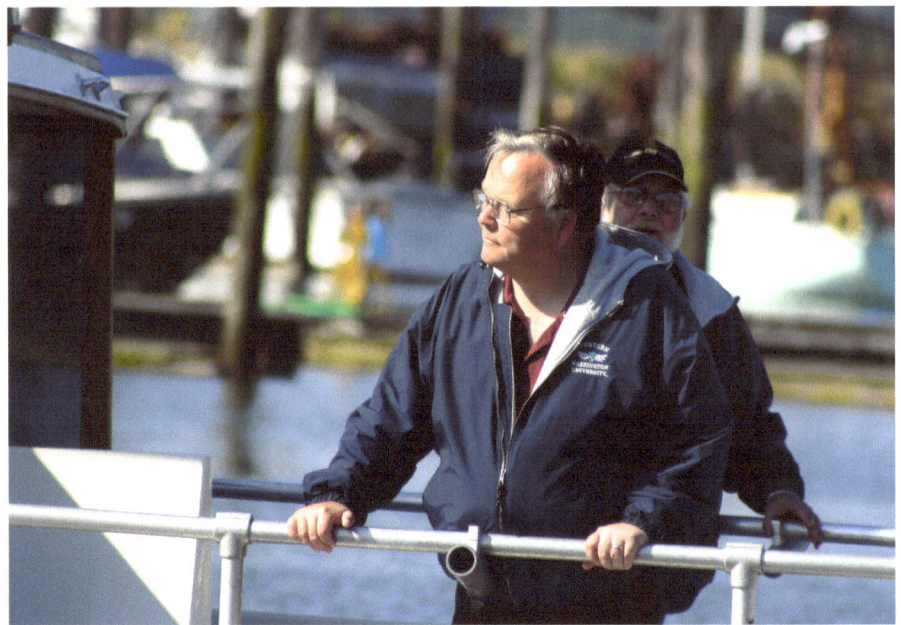

Photo by Colleen Tolva

Dan Tolva returns to port after a fishing adventure.

About the author

Dan Tolva was born on Nov. 3, 1949, in the small fishing village of Ilwaco, Wash., at the mouth of the Columbia River. He arrived two months early along with a twin brother, David, who died after 16 hours.

Tolva weighed but 2 pounds, 3 ounces at birth (He has since made up for that deficit and then some.). He was placed in an incubator to keep him alive, but the oxygen given him damaged his retinas to the point that, according to family lore, he couldn't follow the light of a match when he was little.

The condition was called retrolental fibroplasia at the time, and afflicted thousands of premature "baby boomers" in the years after World War II until it was discovered that too much oxygen in the incubator was to blame. Most victims lost their sight entirely, but Tolva had enough vision to be classified as legally blind.

He was sent to the Washington State School for the Blind in Vancouver at the age of 4, and he graduated from there in 1967, 13 years later. Tolva attended Clark Community College in Vancouver and Western Washington State College in Bellingham. He spent one summer vacation working as a deckhand on his father's 54-foot fishing boat in Alaska. He survived that adventure and went on to earn a bachelor's degree in journalism from Western in December 1972.

Tolva landed a job as a general-assignment reporter at the Vancouver (Wash.) Columbian in May of 1972, eventually covering education, aviation, parks and recreation, and agriculture.

A few years later, he became a copy editor, editing stories, writing headlines and laying out pages for every section of the paper at one time or another. He was also on the board of directors of the paper's credit union as secretary and vice president.

Tolva retired in 2009 after nearly 37 years at The Columbian.

He served as president of the Vancouver Lions Club for two years in the 1980s, played first-chair trumpet and percussion in the Northwest LDS Symphony, produced a television program for Vancouver's cable access channel, and took 10 hours of flying lessons from a series of incredibly brave flight instructors.

In 2008, he composed a symphony, "Columbia Currents: A Musical Journey Down the Great River of the West." He has also taken oboe and guitar lessons, but the less said about the resulting sounds from those endeavors, the better.

In 2014, Tolva produced a video using the music from "Columbia Currents" and photos he and his wife had taken along the Columbia River. Here is what he wrote concerning the video:

"Aside from a few years away at college, I've never lived more than a few miles away from the Columbia River. I was born in the small fishing village of Ilwaco, near the mouth of the Columbia on the Washington side. My dad, uncles, cousins and I fished commercially on the Columbia. I've swam in it, probably polluted it, travelled on and beside it, and always loved *it.*

"In 2008, I wrote a symphony dedicated to the river in five movements, or 'currents: 'Headwaters,' 'Grand Coulee,' 'Hanford Reach,' 'Tributaries,' "The Gorge,' and 'Estuary and Home.' Now, thanks to iMovies, I've married that music to some of the many photos my lovely wife, Colleen, and I have taken over years of traveling up and down the river.

"Now I'm sharing this video on YouTube for your enjoyment. So grab some popcorn and hit the bathroom beforehand, because this show is about 25 minutes long."

(View the YouTube video at: https://www.YouTube.com/watch?v=yQr1spo-dFQ&feature=share.)

In 2015, he wrote "The Possible Life: An autobiography of Dan Tolva." In 2017, he completed "Drawing Power," a collection of pen-and-ink and Adobe Illustrator pictures from the early 1970s on.

Tolva enjoys photography, cooking (but not cleaning up afterwards), and watching TV — especially college football. Anything involving airplanes also grabs his fancy. And he likes boats because they're nautical but nice.

He and his second wife, Colleen, reside in Vancouver, and are active in church and political affairs. Their "blended family" includes five grown children, 12 grandchildren, and three great-grandchildren.

www.ingramcontent.com/pod-product-compliance
Lightning Source LLC
Chambersburg PA
CBHW040321220526
45473CB00009B/2513